Homebirth Cesarean

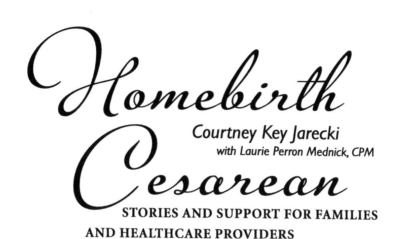

Homebirth

Courtney Key Jarecki
with Laurie Perron Mednick, CPM

Cesarean

STORIES AND SUPPORT FOR FAMILIES AND HEALTHCARE PROVIDERS

Also by Courtney Key Jarecki

Healing from a Homebirth Cesarean
A companion workbook for any mother whose planned out-of-hospital birth ended in the operating room

Printed in the United States of America
First Printing, 2015

ISBN 978-0-9862039-3-0
LCN 2014920275

Incisio Press
Portland, Oregon
www.IncisioPress.com

To Lazadae, your birth changed everything.
You, my daughter, are power and grace.

Dave, thank you for the continued gift of your love.

Success is about so much more than our vaginas.
And a cut in our bellies is not a failure.
—LEAH (2012/HBC, WESTERN U.S.)

And when it could do no more,
it learned, by God, it learned,
there may be endless
ways to open.
—WRITTEN BY SAGE, (2008/HBC, WESTERN U.S.)
FROM THE POEM *Dear Scar,*

Table of contents

The story of the Homebirth Cesarean project

The Homebirth Cesarean project started during my transport to the hospital, in the early morning hours of April 1, 2011. It would be another seven months before the seed of the book came into the world—I opened a new document on my computer, saved it as "homebirth cesarean" and wrote nothing else. I didn't know where to start, but I knew it had to be done.

Laurie is a contributing author and one of the midwives who attended my birth. She and I are proud to offer a first-of-its-kind glimpse into HBC birth, allowing people an opportunity to read perspectives from mothers as well as midwives, doulas, and other birth professionals. This book gives voice to homebirth cesarean women and the birth professionals who support them—many of whom have been silent in the greater birth conversation.

And the book too has birthed something larger than itself—workshops for birth professionals, retreats for HBC mothers, and the groundwork that these conversations continue so that more voices can be heard.

The experience of writing this book and working toward a sustainable conversation about homebirth cesareans has been joyful and painful in equal measures—there have been laughter and tears, frustration and respite, relationships created and strengthened and, in some cases, broken. This book began with one child's need for a cesarean birth, and it has paved the way for thousands of mothers, children, partners, and professionals to reclaim their stories and rename their experiences.

Courtney Key Jarecki —HBC MOTHER

Unearthing a new story

My experience, and the trauma I'm healing from, are directly related to the fact that I planned an out-of-hospital birth and ended up at the hospital. I went from intimate care with a midwife to a hospital I had never visited and people I hadn't met, people who didn't know me at all. I went from client-first support, to caregivers who had a strict set of rules that determined how they treated me. For many of us homebirth cesarean mothers, we are dealing with more than the loss of a vaginal birth. We're struggling with a shattering of our expectations and identities.
—Jo (2012/HBC, Western U.S.)

Homebirth Cesarean defined

Homebirth Cesarean began as a conversation between us: a mother who spiraled from her homebirth dream to the devastating reality of her cesarean birth, and the midwife who served her. Eight months after the birth, we discovered that the nature of our partnership as mother and midwife granted us an opportunity to explore homebirth cesareans from both the client and birth professional perspectives. Until now, no one has interviewed, gathered, and shared these stories or offered practical strategies to support HBC women and families.

A homebirth cesarean (HBC) is not a surgical birth performed at home by midwives. The term, which I first used to define my birth experience with my daughter, describes a planned out-of-hospital birth that ends in cesarean. Even though the word *homebirth* is used, the intended location of the birth can also include freestanding birth centers. Women who choose to birth unassisted, meaning without the help of midwives, can also be homebirth cesarean mothers. HBC may be applied to women who transfer care before labor starts, referred to as pre-labor homebirth cesareans, and to those who transport to the hospital during labor.

By bringing the terms homebirth and cesarean together as a single definition, we honor the homebirth dream that mothers lost during their surgical birth experiences. Through this name, we begin to change the way
we relate to these birth journeys, reaffirming the importance of the HBC
experience in the homebirth and natural birth communities.

> When I first heard the term homebirth cesarean, it seemed inaccurate because I
> had a homebirth that turned cesarean. But the more I thought about it, that was
> exactly the term that was needed. The name gave me a sense of peace I had
> lost after realizing I wasn't a homebirther but refusing to identify as a cesarean
> mom. I wasn't either. I was both. It felt like that term suddenly let me know who
> I was. When I say homebirth cesarean and I see a spark in the other woman's
> eyes, I know she's an HBC mom and we have an instant sisterhood.
> —ALEXIS (2011/HBC, MIDWESTERN U.S.)

Though many women experience sadness, regret, and trauma during their
births, this book focuses specifically on planned out-of-hospital births that
end in cesareans. Homebirth women who were transported to the hospital
and had vaginal births, or hospital birthing women who planned natural
births that ended in cesareans are not featured in these pages, though they
may also suffer devastation and grief from their experiences. The drastic
change in birth venues, the loss of primary relationship-based midwifery
care, and surgical birth are unique factors of the HBC experience that are
explored here.

All mothers deserve an opportunity to share and be validated for the way
that they give birth, no matter the route. Homebirth cesarean mothers
need that chance as well, and that is what this book provides.

Why women choose out-of-hospital birth

Women from all walks of life choose to give birth outside of the hospital.
They are generally well-educated about the differences between the midwifery and Western (allopathic) models of care. Some women decide on
homebirth for one specific reason, such as a fear of hospitals, while others
have a combination of intentions that may include:

- Strong desire for autonomy and privacy

- Family, cultural, social, or historical reasons such as having been born at home themselves or hearing positive out-of-hospital birth stories

- Fear of judgment by hospital staff

- Strong need for control over decisions concerning their bodies and their babies

- Prior negative experiences with hospitals and medical personnel

- Belief that birth is not a medical event for low-risk women

> *I have a severe phobia of needles, doctors, and hospitals, so I knew the hospital was not the right place for me to have a baby.*
> —Cara (2008/HBC, Western U.S.)

> *I was born at home. I loved hearing the story of my birth, and all my life I thought I was going to give birth at home.*
> —Libby (2011/HBC, 2013/VBAC transport; Midwestern U.S.)

> *I wanted to be in an environment where I was comfortable and secure, a place that gave me strength.*
> —Rachel (2009/HBC, Western U.S.)

> *My most powerful birth impressions came from my Peace Corps experience in Micronesia. There was a lot of pride in birth—it was a form of female machismo. I was struck by that and it led me to want that experience.*
> —Carrie (2011/HBC, Western U.S.)

The midwifery model of care

Historically, and across many cultures, women have handed down the art and science of caring for birthing women from midwife to midwife. This model of care is built on the understanding of pregnancy and birth as normal physiological processes. According to Midwives Alliance of North America (MANA), a professional organization for midwives, midwives are responsible for "monitoring the physical, psychological and social wellbeing of the mother throughout the childbearing cycle, and providing the mother with individualized education, counseling, and prenatal care, continuous hands-on assistance during labor and delivery, and postpartum support.[1]" Midwives strive to use technological interventions judiciously, and they refer to physicians the women who require care for higher-risk-medical circumstances, such as gestational diabetes, pre-eclampsia, or post-operative complications. Homebirth midwives typically do not carry malpractice insurance, and women choosing homebirths understand that they must assume responsibility for decision-making and be dedicated to self-care through the prenatal, birth, and postpartum periods.

In addition to the various credentials of midwives, numerous factors determine how midwives structure their care. If a midwife operates in a state where certified professional midwives (CPMs) are illegal, such as Illinois, she may only agree to serve clients with whom she has a strong trusting relationship, and they understand the risk she undertakes in serving them, particularly if complications arise. Further, the midwife may tell clients that in a transport situation, she may not accompany them to the hospital, or may send a doula instead, since she may face legal action initiated by the hospital. In this case, the clients need to have a clear understanding of the benefits of choosing to give birth at home but also the limitations and drawbacks in the event of complications.

Geography and availability of midwives also play a role in the level of care a woman receives. Sherry Dress, a midwife in sparsely populated eastern Oregon, drives hundreds of miles per week to visit her clients, and may be hours away from their homes when labor begins. As their due date approaches, some of her clients choose to stay at Dress's home to give birth, since it is closer to a hospital. When a woman has a homebirth cesarean or other need for intensive postpartum care, Dress will sometimes stay with the family for several days to care for them in case of complications.

On the other hand, urban midwives have the luxury of close proximity to their clients, and they can access a wide range of alternative and Western healthcare providers, plus a greater variety of hospitals. In some places,

---

1   Midwives Alliance of North America. Retrieved September 22, 2014, from http://mana. org/about-midwives/midwifery-model

such as Madison, Wisconsin, the sheer number of homebirth midwives means that women have many options for finding the right care provider for them, which can mean a better ideological and personality fit for the mother and her midwife.

The storytellers

HBC mothers experience both the midwifery and obstetric worlds, encountering firsthand the differences in care. With acute awareness of this disparity, I began the HBC movement as a private Facebook group for mothers and birth professionals. The majority of the interviewees for this book came from that online pool and a few reached us via the Homebirth Cesarean website, www.HomeBirthCesarean.com. Graciously, families and professionals gave their time, sometimes hours, to answer our questions. Most of our full-length interviews took place over the phone, some were in person, some over email, and a few were video chats. As we developed the book, we reached out to the HBC online community asking for people with specific experiences to answer a few questions.

Across the board, women shared their deepest fears and private thoughts, all so their stories could help other families. HBC mother Carol wanted to be interviewed for this book because she loathed the fact that her story is one that people use to discredit homebirths. Midwife Amanda Roe wanted to be part of the birth revolution and ensure that women do not feel so traumatized and bewildered after an HBC.

We searched for recurrent themes in our interviews, like a mother's loss of connection with her birth team after a homebirth cesarean, as well as unique perspectives to truly draw out the many dimensions of HBC. In total, we interviewed more than 250 HBC mothers, partners, midwives, birth workers, mental health professionals, doctors, nurses, and other care providers from around the world.

Some names, locations, and small details have been changed to safeguard the personal or professional identities of families and birth professionals. Children's names have been excluded to protect their privacy. Excerpts from our interviews are the foundation of *Homebirth Cesarean*. The nature of personal reflection shifts viewpoints in dynamic and healing ways. What was true for women during their interviews may be different from how they feel now and how they will feel in years to come. The quotes from mothers are captured moments in time and do not necessarily reveal their current perspective on their birth experience. This is the beauty of forgiveness and acceptance. The same evolution applies to the comments of birth professionals who have learned more about the HBC experience since their interviews and changed the way they work with cesareans.

Special notes about this book

Homebirth Cesarean is not written as an academic work, nor is it a folksy yarn meant to entertain. In writing, we strived for readability and approachability. The intention is to bring HBC families, the natural birth community, and healthcare professionals together to have multilateral conversations about all things HBC.

We recognize that families take many forms, and we have included partners of different sexes and genders, as well as single mothers. We switch gender pronouns throughout the chapters to reflect a diverse population of HBC families.

Breastfeeding can also look different from mother to mother and can be difficult after an HBC. For some women, despite their wishes and best efforts, they may need to use other ways to feed their babies. We understand this can be a gut-wrenching decision, and we honor that by alternately referring to nursing mothers and using a more general description for feeding babies.

We acknowledge that not all homebirth cesareans bring forth living babies, and that these tragic birth stories also require their own understanding and validation. Within the scope of this book, we focus on HBCs that resulted in a living baby.

Pertinent acronyms

CS	Cesarean Section
CPM	Certified Professional Midwife
CNM	Certified Nurse Midwife
RCS	Repeat Cesarean Section
HB	Homebirth
HBC	Homebirth Cesarean
HBAC	Homebirth After Cesarean
ND	Naturopathic Doctor
OCD	Obsessive compulsive disorder
PMADs	Perinatal Mood and Anxiety Disorders
PPD	Postpartum depression
PTSD	Post-traumatic Stress Disorder
VBAC	Vaginal Birth After Cesarean

A guide to this book

Homebirth Cesarean is more than a collection of conversations, stories, scars, and healing. It is about creating a new story—a legend that has previously remained untold. Birth activist Erin Erdman says, "*Homebirth Cesarean* has unearthed a new form of birth that was never before recognized." She is right.

Homebirth Cesarean is designed to follow a mother's journey from pregnancy, through birth, beyond the postpartum year, and continues with the possibility and birth of another child. We show the raw power of birth trauma from home to operating room to back home again, and reveal hopeful resolution pieces for mothers, partners, and birth professionals.

Chapter 1, "The scar we share," is the only memoir in the book. It tells the story of my three-day home labor and transport to the hospital for a cesarean. I carve out my wounds, exposing my shame, isolation, and anger at my inability to birth my baby at home.

Contributing author Laurie Perron Mednick was my midwife during my HBC. Laurie's story follows as a coda as she shares her own route to homebirth cesarean. Laurie reveals her struggles with feelings of self-doubt and impotence when her clients experienced cesareans. These births awoke a deep curiosity within her, driving her to ask more, learn more, and share more with other healthcare professionals about these under-examined yet powerful births.

Claudia Baskind wrote Chapter 9, "Wired for Love." As an HBC mother, she navigates the complex maze of anecdote and research regarding the physical, emotional, developmental, and spiritual effects of surgical birth on children and families. This chapter gives reassurance to mothers and families as they assess the well-being of their children, and offers the middle ground between "my child is doomed" and "my baby is healthy, so it doesn't matter how he was born."

The Appendix contains handouts for HBC families and healthcare providers, including cesarean information sheets that midwives, doulas, and childbirth educators can distribute to clients. For example, Plan C (Appendix A) is an extensive conversation starter and planning tool for families and birth professionals to use as a way to think about the possibility of cesarean. The Appendix items are ordered according to how they first appear in the book.

Homebirth Cesarean is designed to be read from chapter to chapter, as concepts introduced early are referenced throughout. However, we understand that this can be an emotionally heavy read, especially for HBC mothers. We ask that you honor where you are in your healing process. If you feel like a chapter or section may be difficult for you, please leave it for another time. If you do become triggered while reading, a grounding exercise may be beneficial. If you do not have a personal breathing or meditation practice, this simple exercise may be supportive:

Close your eyes and feel your feet on the ground.
Observe your breath.
Take a deep inhale, then exhale.
Feel your breath entering
and exiting your lungs.
Do this several times.
Notice your emotions and thoughts.
Let them be.
Continue to breathe deeply, feeling your feet on the ground.
When you are ready, slowly open your eyes.

Dear Scar,

You new, kissless
lips the surgeon made

through which the slick
tongue of my son's life

took its first taste
of this world. Now empty

of coin or entrance, keeper
of the secret my body

never learned to confess,
your cold lips zipped against

the steel that made you.
It was the midwife who

spoke the sentence:
I was doing it wrong,

I'd never learn to let go.
I'd been rehearsing this

disappointment my entire life,
tracing fingers over

its pressed-in letters
now inscribed: the Shema

across this threshold.
Today, as I kiss my fingers

to you, this door that would not
be blessed, secret seam

where my son and I divided,
your silence is kind. Today I see

an indelible smile stitched
below my stretched-out belly,

the stigmata that says this body
did exactly what it was asked to do.

And when it could do no more,
it learned, by God, it learned,

there may be endless
ways to open.

—WRITTEN BY SAGE (2008/HBC, WESTERN U.S.)

The scar we share

Before the scar

My scar is a red weld once held by staples, a birth site. In its second year, it began to smooth and fade around the edges, the corners raised in a smile. My daughter stares at the scar, asks when she will have one of her own.

The story of my scar stretches out to a time before I joined the homebirth community. I had been working in the corporate world, intent on climbing the ladder even as I failed to find meaning in my work. When the birth world knocked, it was actually a re-knocking, a sound reminiscent of one I'd heard in college when I educated myself on natural birth. The day the corporate world set me free, I accepted a position as a postpartum doula at a Portland, Oregon birth center and began moving forward by returning to my roots. Soon I started a midwifery apprenticeship, steeping my identity in home and birth center births.

Within this proximity of birth, I found myself pregnant, a choice my husband Dave and I had put off for the first eight years of our marriage. But the pregnancy ended in miscarriage; it was a harrowing two-month process that sent fissures through our relationship and caused me to lose faith in my body's ability to sustain and bring life into the world. A month after the miscarriage ended, when I began to let go of the grief, I was pregnant again. Unbeknownst to me, my future scar was gestating.

The dance of mind and body

Throughout my pregnancy, I continued to assist moms and immerse myself in midwifery studies and stories of natural birth. In so doing, I adopted my own opinion of the birth process—namely, that labor is about surrender, acceptance, and releasing control.

Paradoxically, I was convinced that my understanding of birth would make me an ideal laboring mother. When I met with my midwives, Laurie and Kim, for our prenatal appointments, there were three midwives in the room. We conversed as peers, swapped stories back and forth, even shrugged off the possibility of transport, and the word cesarean was never mentioned. Why would it be? In my mind, cesareans only happened to women who worked against birth's natural flow. Birth, however painful and tornado-like, would unfold in a natural fashion for me.

I visualized where my baby would be born, imagined her first cries and breast crawl, prepped Dave on why we would wait to cut the umbilical cord, and explained how I'd use my placenta medicinally. I allowed myself to be swept up in the romance of homebirth and whenever I felt that I was delving too far into magical thinking about creating the ideal birth, I relied on my clinical understanding that my body was designed to give birth.

When labor started—March 29, two hours shy of midnight—I moved from our bed to the couch and revisited the supplies I'd set out for myself over the course of the previous week: the calming flower essences, waterproof pads, and instructions I'd written down for the midwives. Looking back, my innocence is astounding, my hope heartbreaking.

When the darkness comes
The first full day of labor became the first full night, then the second full day. Throughout the process, I secretly congratulated myself on how well I was handling the contractions, actively creating the experience I wanted. There was no doubt that I would continue to dance through the process. Toward the middle of the second day, I felt my labor shift. With the onset of rectal pressure, my brain re-engaged with the clinical aspects of what was happening.

The baby is descending. I must be six or seven centimeters by now. I'm nearing transition.

On my hands and knees in the birth tub, I told Dave to call the midwives. Never mind that my self-assessments were off, that my baby was still high in my pelvis and I was nowhere near transition.

At the back end of this false awareness, hours after Laurie and Kim arrived, as the second day became the second night, and the clock began to tip toward day three, I agreed to my first cervical check. After all, labor should have progressed by now. Something was off. Was it my body? Was it my assessments?

Lying flat on my bed, deep in the midst of intense back labor, I felt myself sink under the weight of not only the past few days but of the previous nine months, and of the two-plus years during which I'd been supporting the births of other women. As Laurie slipped her gloved fingers inside my body, I could tell by her expression that something wasn't right.

She looked off to the side, choosing her words carefully. "Your cervix is soft," she said, adding that she felt the baby's head, and that I was only three centimeters dilated. She used the term *constriction ring* and described it as a tight band of tissue, like a rubber band around a broccoli stalk.

The weight of my homebirth dream deepened. I trembled under it. My mind kicked in again.

Two full days, three centimeters. Why is my body failing? Where's the birth I deserved?

After Dave coaxed me from the dark pit I was sinking into, we tried a new labor position. I dropped in a crouch, falling into his arms, my body spilling into his lap. We found a new rhythm, agreed that my cervix was opening now, convinced ourselves—falsely again—that labor was transitioning, wishing more than anything to enact our hopeful wills against desperation. We saw what appeared to be the first glimpses of bloody show, a sure sign that we were moving in the right direction. We were more than hopeful now—gleeful, present, aware. Then Kim took a flashlight to examine the substance on the floor between my feet. There was no blood, only meconium.

My clinical brain clicked into overdrive, tumbling and twisting in on itself with numbers and figures and words.

Water broken for fifty hours. Three centimeters. Constriction ring. Meconium. Failure.

Descent

When Dave asked Kim if it was time to talk about "other options," I knew what he was implying. He wanted to say *transport, hospital, doctor.* Even without him saying those words, the notion stung, toppled upon the pile of other words building in my head.

Water broken. Constriction ring. Meconium. Other options.

When Laurie and Kim huddled to devise a new plan, I slipped into the bathroom to wipe the meconium oozing between my legs. It was thick and dark as pitch, giving off a smell of something earthen and dead, like an animal buried beneath autumn mulch.

Fifty hours. Meconium. Hospital. Something dying inside me.

In this spiraling moment I began to float outside of myself. I left my body, hovered somewhere near the ceiling and looked down on the swollen woman alone near the sink. A hump of human flesh, a presence coming face to face with a sudden awareness that would hit her like a jolt. The woman near the sink had miscarried in this bathroom a year earlier. The woman near the sink was losing contact with the baby inside of her. The woman near the sink would need a surgeon's scalpel to complete her birth.

When I came back into my body, I gathered as many splintered pieces of myself as I could and walked to the kitchen. Laurie and Kim were ready to share their plan, but I didn't let them speak.

Meconium. Other options. Something dying. A scar being born.

I told them we needed to go, and before they could summon a word between them, I added that the baby would be born in the operating room. Forget the positive possibilities they quickly threw at me—an IV, epidural, some rest. "Operating room," I said because I knew what I knew—that I was a failure, that I'd miscarried one child and would be unable to vaginally birth another. I tuned them out along with the music of my own body, the natural birth rhythm, however disoriented it was, that had become the past three days.

Changing states

The room turned wobbly then, as if the magnitude of my decision shot ripples through the entire house. Dave slipped into his own form of despair, grew distant and dark, drifted away into an angry, shutdown state of denial. He didn't want to pack, wouldn't bring the laptop, refused to accept that we'd be staying a few days in the hospital. He clung to the remaining vapors of the homebirth dream that, for me, had already evaporated.

Laurie and Kim split off as well. Laurie stood in the kitchen, making a phone call to the hospital, while Kim tracked through the hallway, upstairs, then back down, trying to gather things for me to pack. I was alone again, still contracting, still very much going through the action of labor. Unaided and forgotten, I was down to my last reserves, lacking comfort or physical support, no hand to hold, no body to cradle me through the spasms. Yet I sprang to attention and began barking orders, arguing with Dave about what to pack, instructing Kim where to find this and that. And our dogs—so present and aware during the entire labor—suddenly they were trembling from the energy as well. They paced as Dave paced and watched as he called our friend in the middle of the night to come and take care of them. They felt the ripples we were casting.

Laurie said the midwife at the hospital we were transporting to was the best, but as she spoke, I couldn't bring myself to care. Could she not see my anger? My grief? My certainty of how this birth would end? I didn't want her kindness, didn't think I deserved it. Her words, meant to be supportive, had the opposite effect—they grated on my psyche.

When Kim helped me out to our van, I spewed my self-loathing at her. "I'm worthless," I said. "I fucked up my first pregnancy. Now this." Deep down, I wanted to tell her how scared I was, but that quiet, revealing voice stayed buried. She helped me into the car, made sure I was as comfortable as possible, handed me a water bottle, then walked to her car and led our procession to the hospital. What I needed more than anything was for someone to hold me, to sit with me and let me unravel, to tell me I was brave.

By the time Dave took the driver's seat, the smell of meconium became a foul, fierce reality, a putrid scent that infiltrated my senses. I could taste it, feel it. I equated the morning's darkness with its color. As the car bumped along and the smell crawled up the very middle of my body, I was certain my baby was dead.

Of dreams and visions

Our daughter's name came to me just after conception, before I had taken a pregnancy test. Her name and sex were known without a doubt, all because I'd dreamt that I had a tray of lasagna in the oven. From the word lasagna came Lazadae, a girl never needing an ultrasound to prove she was in there. A dream both Dave and I trusted with the whole of our hearts.

But there were other dreams I shied from, tried to ignore, to turn off, to pretend were nothing more than random images. Dreams in which strangers handed me my baby, where the child arrived suddenly, taken from my body and dropped into my arms. I shared these with Laurie and Kim, but we never sought to explore them. We passed them off as pregnancy dreams, the mind processing the events of the day.

At the hospital in the labor room, when the fetal monitor showed Lazadae's beating heart, I was neither relieved nor grateful. Instead, my lungs held the hospital's stale air for an abnormal length of time, then released it in a grunt. While I was unable to properly breathe, Lazadae responded with heart decelerations. She and I were working as a team again, alerting the hospital staff they needed to prep for surgery, that a vaginal birth would not happen, even as they tried to convince me otherwise. The dream of a stranger taking my baby from my body was about to happen.

Soon people began to listen, to hear us, to acknowledge our truth. Papers came looking for signatures. Everyone circled to explain what was happening. I didn't care to hear the steps. I wanted to move toward the conclusion. And within the preparation and motion, Dave and I lost one last opportunity to be alone together, to acknowledge what was happening, and what was about to happen. I was voiceless, shut down, as far removed from myself as possible. I floated away again, saw my gowned frame from outside my body contracting next to the bed.

If there was a savior to be found, it was Liz, the hospital nurse midwife Laurie had mentioned before we left home. Liz spoke clearly and plainly and met me where I was with an open face encompassed by a halo of white light. She walked me to the operating room, held my hand as I contracted again, stayed near me at all times—the perfect birth attendant in those moments of overwhelming need and grief.

The meconium was pouring out of me now. Before sitting on the operating table, I kicked my underwear out of sight, not wanting anyone to see, certain I wouldn't have been able to handle the looks on their faces when they saw the physical evidence of what was happening inside my body.

Dave entered the operating room, masked and gowned. I remember glancing at him, but nothing more. Later Dave would tell me he and I held eye contact during the entire surgery, describing a moment that, for him, was one of the most intimate exchanges we ever shared. I remember none of it. I was out of my body, saw and heard nothing beyond my own thoughts. No blue drape inches from my face. No smell of burning flesh as the surgeon sliced my womb. No tugging as they pulled my uterus outside my body and wrapped it in a warm towel. I did not respond to Dave's loving touch. I was gone, my spirit traveling to unknowable places, searching for my daughter to bring her back to the world alive.

A cavern opened, forced by human hands, and we were separated, pulled in opposite directions. At 7:04 on the morning of April Fools' Day, a stranger in surgical scrubs lifted my surprise breech baby to the sky, an offering to the world. Her long legs were piked to her chest, feet touching her ears. My body went toward her. I could see an imprint of myself floating, following closely as she was carried across the room. Unable to bear the secret of my stillbirth, I told Liz I knew it all along. She asked me to hear the cries, but I only heard silence. "You're lying to me," I said. "My baby is dead."

It took Dave placing his hand on her blue chest for her to pink up and for me to understand that she was alive. Her cries, loud and long, pierced my nightmare. It was his hand that allowed me to witness her as a living, beautiful daughter. Dave nuzzled her underneath his scrubs and carried her to me, whispering, *Lazadae*.

I held her tight as they wheeled us to the recovery room where Laurie and Kim waited. Relief, disbelief, gratitude, and ecstasy swirled as I tried to talk through the thickness of drugs and fatigue. I wanted to ask, *What happened? Why was she born this way? What does this mean for us now?*

Still clinging

Little did I know that the hospital stay, a bubble of safety for us, would be the calmest and most peaceful two days of my postpartum year. My attending nurses were homebirth supporters and were sorry I'd had a cesarean. With the exception of an orthopedic surgeon who threatened months in a full-body harness to treat Lazadae's hip dysplasia caused from her breech position, we were respected by the hospital staff. Lazadae and I were able to begin integrating our birth experience as we snuggled under a fuzzy blue blanket brought from home. I used that blanket to hide hospital details in photos sent to family and friends. I was left to rest, care for my baby, and internalize my fears and anxiety without interruption.

I knew something was wrong with breastfeeding, but I could not yet figure out what it was. Two lactation consultants told me everything was normal, and it was Laurie who gave me permission to start pumping before a problem was identified. Finally, someone was validating my unease and doubts. Her acknowledgement was significant because, even if she didn't think something was actually wrong, she allowed me to try to fix it.

On my last day in the hospital, I looked at my stapled stomach in the bathroom mirror and my drug-induced fog began to lift. I saw myself broken. My infuriation swelled, growing tighter and immense. My athletic body that used to do everything I asked of it was now unable to move without shearing pain. I could barely wipe myself after going to the bathroom, and putting my own shoes on for the car ride home was out of the question.

I wanted to film Dave welcoming Lazadae to her new home, but the walk from the driveway up the four front steps and into the living room took my breath away. It felt like the house itself was holding its breath, awaiting our return. The heat had been left on high from the labor and the air held the smell of abandonment and dread. My unused homebirth supplies mocked me from the living room corner. The sadness caused me to lose my balance. I turned the camera off and cried. Dave was holding Lazadae and no one was holding me. We were alone, without support.

A few hours later, I started shaking—violent full-body shakes that caused me to lose bladder control and clutch the walls. I was afraid I would fall to the ground and split open at the incision. The bed shook when I trembled and Dave held me with one hand as he cradled Lazadae in the other. A pool of urine spread between my legs.

Triggers, fears, and the road toward healing

The onset of evening held a dark power over me. I felt crushed by the mere thought of sleeping sitting up, although the surgery left me no other option. My experience destroyed me, leaving me violated and defenseless. For weeks I would not allow friends to see me; Dave met them in the driveway to collect their gifts of food, apologizing. I retreated and cut off all connections except with those who were directly able to support my breastfeeding efforts or Lazadae's hip dysplasia. My humiliation at failing to give birth vaginally caused me to feel less than human and unworthy of love.

Guilt and shame strangled my mind, trying to convince me that Lazadae did not want me to be her mother, that she knew she deserved a safer passage into her life. But I loved my daughter, and somewhere inside, I knew these thoughts weren't true. I held her every moment I could and explained the emotions I was having. I told her that I needed to feel this way so I could be a better mama for her. I apologized over and over. Her presence was the only joy in my life.

Every day and night Dave syringe-fed Lazadae donated milk while I sat in the glider and pumped empty breasts. As she sucked the milk from his finger, she turned her head toward me, always keeping me close. Our bond was strong. Lazadae's determination, strength, and love kept me on this earth. Her bright eyes, open heart, and old soul held my broken spirit.

Laurie and Kim made several extra home visits for two weeks after the birth, then regular postpartum care resumed. I felt comfort and confusion in their presence. Though I was invited to process the birth with them, there was an unspoken story between us, something no one wanted to talk about. My mind was in a state of chaos, both frenzied and vacant, and I was unable to ask for what I needed because I wasn't sure what would help.

They lacked the knowledge to help me navigate my cesarean recovery. Laurie did not know how to help me stand up, roll over, or cough without pain. When I asked Kim to examine my incision, she was hesitant and nervous, saying she usually avoided looking at them. They did not know why I was trembling, and they had no advice on how to remove my incision bandages. Their inability to provide me with basic information and resources felt like a dismissal of the sacrifice I'd made to give birth.

For the next six months, everything took me back to the cesarean. I could not make milk because I had a cesarean. There were nights when Lazadae slept without me because I had a cesarean. Every time I warmed milk from another mother and slipped a feeding tube between my breast and Lazadae's mouth, I was reminded of my cesarean. I felt brutalized because I could not provide basic care for my daughter. At times, I wanted my life to end because I had a cesarean.

How could I continue with midwifery studies if I could not give birth vaginally? Feeling like a black cloud of bad luck, I was unable to imagine women wanting my support as they planned their homebirths. My whole world, identity, and belief system were shattered, and my physical, emotional, and spiritual bodies were crashing down around me. My postpartum depression manifested as loneliness and isolation, and I believed I would never heal. I was embarrassed, angry, and in denial. Driving in the car, something I did often for Lazadae's hip appointments, was a trigger for my PTSD. I had anxiety every time I had to search for, coordinate, and pick up donor breast milk, a 20-hour a week task. Keeping Lazadae off formula was a matter of life and death in my mind, and I gave everything to find her breast milk every day.

While Dave slipped back into his career responsibilities and compartmentalized the birth, distractions fundamental to my survival kicked in. I researched alternatives to a full-body harness to help set Lazadae's hips. I learned to navigate the complicated milk-sharing community. I scheduled appointments with lactation consultants, body workers, and therapists. For 18 weeks, I tried everything from hypnotherapy to prescription drugs to try to induce milk production. These tasks were necessary, demanded my focus, and served as life-saving complications, but they did not help me heal. If it had not been for my inability to make milk, I would have been left without something towards which to direct my manic energy. Without that responsibility to focus on, I would have plummeted into a darkness so deep that I'm not sure I would have been able to pull myself out.

Feedback to my midwives

As the weeks went by, questions bubbled forth: Where was the support when I needed it? Why did my midwifery bookshelf not contain one text about cesarean recovery? Why was the only person who knew enough about cesarean a midwife friend who herself had had one?

For months, I composed an email to Laurie and Kim about their postpartum care. It began as a letter of anger that morphed into one of sad betrayal, and it always ended by asking them not to respond; I did not want to hear what they had to say. It was not until I began to forgive myself that I could compose a letter worth sending. (See Chapter 7 for the email I sent to Laurie and Kim.)

Their reply was swift and kind. Eight months after the birth, we met at their office for a two-hour conversation. I learned of their own heartbreak and grief, and they shared how they understood that their support had not been enough. We talked through what future mothers whose homebirths turn cesarean might need and why midwifery was not supporting these types of births. I knew that homebirth was about empowerment, and I needed to understand why midwifery was not empowering mothers to accept that all forms of birth are valid, even those that include a surgeon's knife.

Laurie's story

I decided to become a midwife in 1994, my junior year as a premedical student at the University of Vermont, while recovering from surgery that had removed a malignant thyroid tumor. Lying in bed with a painful scar on my throat that rendered me speechless, I knew that not only had my health changed course dramatically but the arc of my career had veered in an unexpected direction. I had become deeply disillusioned by the medical system I'd engaged for treatment of my cancer, and I could not imagine becoming yet another doctor with an inability to provide *health*care. Seeking information on the cause of my tumor, my doctors simply reassured me that I could be cut open and the malignancy removed. I knew then that my future held a calling that would cultivate curiosity and value collaboration between patients and providers. After graduating from college, I moved west and became a labor doula in Berkeley, California, serving immigrant women. My husband and I moved to Portland, Oregon, in 1999, and I immediately began training to become a childbirth educator.

I gave birth at home to my first son, Samuel, in 2003, and the following year began studies at Birthingway College of Midwifery. I was delighted to become an apprentice to the midwife who served me during my own birth, and I was soon assisting births in homes and at a birth center. The next four years moved at a rapid-fire pace as I attended births, worked part-time as a childbirth educator, and completed midwifery school. In 2007, just weeks after graduation, I gave birth at home to my second son, Sage. I continued working at the birth center and also joined two classmates in forming our own midwifery practice.

Time and time again, I saw how shell-shocked women were after being transported to the hospital for a cesarean. I was surprised by the depth of grief these mothers experienced, and I knew that many of them withheld candid feedback from me. During case reviews, my fellow midwives and I were at a loss as to how we could have better served these women. I struggled to maintain balance between caring for the intensive needs of the new cesarean family while still seeing my other clients and nurturing myself and my own growing family.

The intimate nature of homebirth midwifery is such that I come to care deeply for my clients, and their hopes for birth become my hopes as well. Whenever that hope was obliterated by a cesarean, I felt the gravity of their loss, yet I lacked the experience and skills to help them navigate their grief. As a new midwife, I worried whether my undeveloped intuition had missed an important signal that could have helped the mother give birth at home. After a cesarean, my own need for emotional protection prevented me from asking questions of my clients that would invite honest feedback. Walking with clients through difficult births is heart-wrenching work, and I did not yet have the wisdom to process my own feelings about homebirth cesareans. The result was that I carried layers of guilt, uncertainty, and unresolved grief into each birth I attended, and this baggage sometimes felt like a wound that never completely healed.

Attending Courtney's birth

I met Courtney in 2010 while caring for mutual clients, and we bonded over sleepless nights with laboring women. When she first became pregnant, Courtney hired my partner Kim and me to provide care for her. After a devastating miscarriage, Courtney came back to us when she became pregnant again.

When I arrived at Courtney's home after receiving her labor call, I found her working beautifully with her contractions. Her husband was perched nearby and the dogs were draped on the couch. I left Courtney and Dave to work alone together for the night, and I returned the following afternoon with Kim when Courtney's labor had progressed and she needed more support. The night wore on as Courtney's contractions intensified and her energy dwindled. We took turns rubbing her back, feeding her, and helping her move into various positions. I was just weeks away from giving birth to my third child; my own back was begging for relief through the darkest hours. After I lay down for a brief nap, Kim woke me to say that she was seeing meconium.

We all agreed that transporting to the hospital was the next logical step, since labor was not progressing and the meconium was a possible sign of fetal distress. While Kim helped Courtney gather her things and monitored the baby's heart rate, I called the hospital to arrange care with the nurse midwives. I needed Liz, the nurse midwife on duty, to comprehend the depth of anguish that this transport would cause Courtney, and I enlisted her in smoothing out the edges of a devastating situation by asking her to stay with them throughout the birth. Courtney requested that Kim accompany her and Dave to the hospital. I would stay behind to clean their home and drain the birth tub before I met them there.

I arrived at the hospital an hour later as Courtney was departing for the operating room. Dave was waiting for the nurse to escort him, and he voiced his fears about what this cesarean meant for Courtney—she would never be the same again, the Courtney he knew was already gone, both emotionally and spiritually. I understood what he meant, and I shared the same concern.

As Dave had predicted, the woman who came back to the labor room dazed, drugged, and exhausted was not the woman who had eagerly begun her labor a few days before. I stayed until Courtney and Lazadae nursed and were ready for sleep, then quietly said my goodbyes to the new family. I was exhausted, hungry, emotionally spent, and needed to be with my own family, but I also understood when Courtney asked me to stay a bit longer. Eventually, I departed, promising to return the following day.

The next days were a blur for me, as I knew they were for Courtney and her family. With two young sons who missed my attention, I struggled to catch up on sleep. I felt deeply saddened by Courtney's unexpected cesarean, but I now had the insight I'd lacked as a new midwife to appreciate that cesareans sometimes need to happen despite the best efforts of the mother, baby, and the birth team.

When I returned to the hospital, I found Courtney frantically sorting out the conflicting breastfeeding advice of nurses and lactation consultants, and I gently reassured her that her intuition superseded the opinions of the hospital staff. Once Courtney was discharged from the hospital, her need for support was even greater. Courtney and I spoke by phone frequently throughout those early days, and I saw her in her home many times in the next few weeks. I felt torn by the demands of caring for Courtney and for the other moms who had recently given birth. At times, I was discouraged to see that the care I was giving Courtney had little impact—I could not help her enough, Kim could not help her enough, nobody could.

No amount of sitting with Courtney on her bed listening to her sorrow and grief seemed to lessen her pain. Communication with her was difficult during the early weeks as she made panicked phone calls requesting my presence but then seemed unsatisfied when I spent time at her home. When I tentatively encouraged her to process the birth, Courtney retreated, much to my relief. Dave seemed angry when I visited, and I was not sure if he was angry with me or just plain angry. As the weeks went by, Kim and I continued our postpartum visits, yet we both sensed that there was a barrier between Courtney and us. Plus, I needed to make an emotional shift toward compartmentalizing Courtney's experience so I could look ahead to my own birth.

In hindsight, I see the need for prenatal conversations that involved more than just filling out a hospital transport plan. If Courtney and I had delved deeply into the unhappy topic of unexpected outcomes, and specifically about cesarean birth, she might have felt more prepared when it did happen. Or perhaps if we had made a comprehensive postpartum care plan that included resources and information for partners, she and Dave might have had time to digest the possibility of needing more care after her birth, and rallied their friends and family beforehand. I also see where I could have better handled those early postpartum conversations. Instead of circumnavigating Courtney's turbulent emotional and mental landscape, I should have addressed her needs for processing her birth and given her written resources for mental health care. I didn't yet understand that my inability to guide Courtney on post-operative care meant that she had nobody who could look, assess, and mentor her on self-care.

The next chapter
In my practice, I see clients for their last visit eight weeks after they give birth. I finalize my care with them and allow for closure of their child-bearing year. Some of those visits are truly bittersweet and lovely; spending most of our time reflecting together on the birth, I elicit feedback, and the families look ahead to the next phase of their journey. Other last visits are chaotic, with little time for birth-processing and closure—there are toddlers needing snacks and mothers rushing to pick up older siblings at school.

When birth does not proceed according to a woman's expectations, those final visits are difficult for both the client and me. Fear, disappointment, confusion, and grief sit in the room with us. I can almost picture the thought bubbles over each person's head. The mom is speculating: *Did I disappoint her? Does she think I'm a failure? Why didn't she know how to help me?* Meanwhile, the midwife is wondering: *Does she hate me? Does she think I failed her? What will she tell others about me?*

The final visit comes early in a woman's new life as a fledgling mother, and she has not had enough time to fully digest her birth experience, even in the best of circumstances. When I gently open the door to discussing a client's birth experience and how they feel about it, they sometimes are unwilling or just not quite ready.

Courtney's final appointment followed the mold of the awkward last visit. She seemed shell-shocked and was unable to share her feelings or offer feedback. While this was not surprising, given the nature of her birth and postpartum transition, it was unfortunate since I wanted clarity about how she perceived her experience and reassurance that she thought my care fulfilled her needs.

I gave birth to my third son that summer, six weeks after Courtney's birth, and, snuggling Kestrel in my arms, I wondered if Courtney was able to enjoy those sweet moments of her own. It was then that I realized how badly I wanted that for her. It was the first opportunity I took to acknowledge that I was terribly disappointed that she had such a difficult birth experience and that she was unable to produce enough milk to sustain her baby. In the weeks before, and then after my own birth, I needed to separate Courtney's birth from mine, and I couldn't fully sink into the weight of my grief regarding her birth experience until my own birth story was written. I wanted to call her, to invite her over for tea, but I was not sure my efforts would be welcome. I was also reluctant to reach out because I felt there was such a disparity in our births. While I did not feel guilty for the birth I experienced, I recognized that there is a certain unfairness in labor and birth outcomes, and I had drawn the lucky straw repeatedly. I knew that I would be unable to share with Courtney my own birth story at a time when she was still grieving for her own.

Eight months after Courtney's birth, Kim and I received an email from her, obviously well thought out and heartfelt, requesting a meeting with us. The timing was fortuitous, since I had just encountered Jenny, a previous client who had had a cesarean birth.

Jenny's birth experience
Jenny was one of the first clients I served in the final year of my apprenticeship. She and her husband were exuberant about becoming parents, and she was eager to greet the work of labor. At her 36-week home visit, we discussed the usual plans for hospital transport and answered their few questions about transferring should the need arise. Optimistic and confident by nature, Jenny focused on preparing for the birth that she wanted. I, too, was caught up in her excitement, and I didn't know how to present unwanted outcomes without dampening her enthusiasm.

Four weeks later, Jenny's labor presented her with a baby in distress and in need of an immediate cesarean. The look on her exhausted and bewildered face after her cesarean revealed the beginning of a dark and traumatic recovery period.

In the weeks following her birth, Jenny did not want to talk about her experience. She seemed depressed, shocked, and in need of grief counseling, yet unable to initiate contact with the referrals I gave her. She felt blindsided by how her labor unfolded, clearly unable to consider the possibility that she could have needed a cesarean.

I did not see Jenny until almost five years later, when fate brought us together in a random encounter. Coming face to face in a narrow, noisy room filled with preschoolers, Jenny stared at me, tilting her head in thought as she considered how we might have known each other. With my child tugging me by the hand out the door, and my sleeping baby beginning to rouse in my arms, she calmly stated that my voice was familiar to her, and she knew me from somewhere. I imagined that perhaps she had blocked her memory of me, and I quietly affirmed that I knew her too, while wondering what her reaction would be if she recalled who I was. The thought of triggering raw memories for her prevented me from revealing our shared past, and I quickly left.

That was the same week I received the email from Courtney, and I knew that these two incidents signified that I had some work to do.

The meeting

Many fears and insecurities arose in the days after I read Courtney's email. My heart told me that I had given her good care, and that the trauma and grief surrounding her birth were hers alone. I was not sure that anyone could have shielded her from her devastating experience. I wanted to avoid this difficult conversation altogether, and I defensively recalled the many long hours I'd spent in her home during and after her birth. It was such a jumbled stew of feelings, but one clear thought rose to the top: regardless of how much care I had given Courtney, the fact remained that she had needed more—or different—care. I realized that she did not want to give me feedback about what a terrible midwife I was. She needed to tell me how she felt about my care.

The day of the meeting, Kim and I braced ourselves for the uncomfortable conversation ahead. We reviewed Courtney's chart and discussed how we felt about her birth and postpartum care. I considered where to sit in the room, since being directly across from Courtney felt too close and vulnerable—I wanted the comfort of distance if she was angry. I also reminded myself that my job was to truly listen to her without defensiveness, and I acknowledged that my own feelings were separate and valid as well.

As I listened to Courtney, I found myself imagining each one of my prior HBC clients sitting in her seat, sharing similar feelings. Yet these women had never contacted me with feedback, never stopped by to say hello, and rarely appeared at the new-moms' groups or homebirth family picnics. In fact, they had become nearly invisible.

The silence of HBC mothers

I now know that during their postpartum care, HBC women are often reluctant to share critical feedback with their midwives, and instead they might seem quiet, "shut down," or simply polite. If a woman has negative feelings about her experience with her midwives, she will probably go through the motions of receiving care and then sever communication after that. Midwives, unless they actively seek this crucial feedback, may not know how a client feels, and the opportunity for growth and resolution is lost.

In conferences and midwifery gatherings, homebirth cesareans are rarely discussed and never celebrated. Perhaps some midwives feel that cesareans are a reflection of their own inadequacies. Is it a blow to a midwife's ego? Is it that midwives fail to appreciate the depth of grief and trauma resulting from HBCs? Is it just too uncomfortable to seek honest feedback from clients?

As I mulled over my history of serving HBC families, it dawned on me that there was a need for midwives and other healthcare providers to learn more, to find out how women felt about these births, and how they were affected by their experiences. During the meeting with Courtney, I proposed that we collaborate on an article; she countered with a book. With Courtney's perspective as a former student midwife and an HBC mama, and my experience as a midwife, we felt that we were in a unique position to bring HBC into the light, and soon afterwards, we began this collaboration.

Untitled

And after three days he cried
Mama.
Mama, I cannot come to you.
Mama, I am so tired.
Mama, please reach in,
*   please send help.*
Mama,
I cannot finish the journey alone.

And in the wee hours of the third day
she lay down her ego,
she lay down her pride,
she poured her tears on the earth.

And she cut a hole in her own flesh
to do what all mothers do—
that which must be done.

She rent her dreams to make a way,
and she brought her sweet baby home.

—Written by Ann (2011/HBC, Midwestern U.S.)

Chapter 2

Considering cesarean

Women planning homebirths are completely unprepared for a cesarean birth, and it sideswipes them in a way that is devastating. Yes, the physical experience is shocking, but psychologically, it is really unexpected. Often, cesarean has never really entered their realm of possibility. Partly, this is because home-birth midwives don't feel comfortable preparing them for that outcome. Cesarean birth is a forbidden topic, and people worry they may plant seeds that might contribute to that outcome. There's a subtle message that if you really trust in the process, then it's all going to go okay. A lot of women invest in that, and that's good, but it leaves them totally unprepared for a whole potential avenue that their life might take.

—Brooke Noli, counselor and certified birth doula, Western U.S.

No matter how a pregnant woman envisions her labor proceeding, it may be nearly impossible for her to imagine being transported to the hospital, completely exhausted and scared, and consenting to a cesarean birth. For many women, the very act of choosing out-of-hospital birth means they are resisting the pervasive cultural message that birth is inherently dangerous and scary, and they are opposing medical interventions routinely offered in the hospital. Perhaps the idea of giving birth by cesarean is so terrifying that any potential conversations about it are off-limits in their minds. Some women simply find the chances of needing a cesarean so unlikely that exploring the possibility seems senseless.

For their part, birth teams vary greatly in how much time they devote to discussing and planning for a transport and its accompanying decisions and interventions. Some midwives or doulas may offer few opportunities to fully explore the topic, while others openly and frequently discuss planning for potential birth complications requiring a hospital transport. Most often, however, the discussion of cesarean birth is ignored, glossed over, or patently dismissed. When birth professionals fail to address cesarean birth, it can be because they are uncomfortable with handling the topic, or they might reject the possibility that it could happen to their client. They may also focus on only positive birth scenarios for fear of manifesting unwanted outcomes.

Yet midwives we interviewed estimate that as many as half of their labor transports end in cesareans. When midwives and their clients neglect to consider, and make a comprehensive plan for a potential cesarean, the resulting shock and grief for HBC women can be devastating. As part of prenatal education, women and their partners need to understand that transport to the hospital means that a cesarean birth is a strong possibility.

This chapter examines the barriers that discourage women from accepting the possibility of a homebirth cesarean; explores the roles of the midwife, doula, and childbirth educator in preparing families; and describes some of the tools that birth professionals can use to guide mothers through difficult conversations about the real possibility of a surgical birth.

Prenatal conversations with midwives
Homebirth midwives work hard to build open, trusting relationships with their clients, but even so, the majority of HBC mothers report that their midwives never specifically discussed cesarean as a possible outcome during their prenatal care. If the conversation around cesarean birth is minimized or entirely absent, how can women understand the midwife's role in the hospital throughout a cesarean, what options might be available in the operating room, or how postpartum recovery and breastfeeding will be different after a surgical birth? As birth advocate Erin Erdman says, "It's difficult enough to be in labor, then to have a complication. Moms shouldn't be worrying about what their midwives will think of them if they transport, what will happen at the hospital, the relationship between their midwives and the doctor, or if their midwives are going to stick around during a cesarean. Moms should know all that ahead of time."

> The truth is that cesareans are sometimes unavoidable, yet I don't remember my midwife talking about this possibility. Looking back, I don't know if this is something she failed to do or if she did bring it up and I was completely resistant. I do know we didn't have real conversations about it.
> —ANN (2011/HBC, MIDWESTERN U.S.)

I felt informed, aware, and prepared for what was going to happen in the home. The hospital was where the preparation stopped.
—DAVE, PARTNER OF COURTNEY (2011/HBC, WESTERN U.S.)

My midwives saw me as someone who was really knowledgeable, which I was. They assumed I knew a lot, and I did. They provided enough general information for me then, because I had no idea I would have needed to know more than that. All their discussions gave a superficial take on the hospital. There really wasn't a conversation of "this may be really hard for you to conceive of, but if you are in the hospital, this is what is going to happen. When I say we aren't going to be in charge of your care anymore, or that there might be interventions that you have a say in and ones you don't have a say in, this is what I specifically mean."
—RACHEL (2009/HBC, WESTERN U.S.)

My midwife said we should think about transport, but she never mentioned the word "cesarean." I was very closed off to considering it. She probably could have brought it up again or pushed me to think about it. It was definitely my worst fear.
—ALICIA (2009/HBC, 2011/HBAC; WESTERN U.S.)

It probably won't happen to you

I made a vow when I was in labor that I would never lie to pregnant women again by giving them all these rigid rules around birth—your body was made to give birth, if you relax you will have a vaginal birth. These natural childbirth slogans, while inspirational and positive, create shame and failure for women whose births don't go as planned.
—PAM ENGLAND, AUTHOR AND FOUNDER OF BIRTHING FROM WITHIN, WESTERN U.S.

Many of the women we interviewed noted that when they wanted to discuss cesarean, their midwives reassured them that a cesarean wouldn't happen or was very unlikely. Or, if the midwife initiated the conversation, it was premised with: "Well, it probably won't happen to you but...." When a woman receives blind reassurance that a cesarean will not be her reality, she disregards the possibility, sees the details as irrelevant, and pushes her fears into the dark corners of her mind.

One of the biggest challenges for birth professionals is to walk the line between instilling confidence in a mother about the birthing process and conveying the very real possibility that she may require a cesarean to safely birth her baby. In order to serve women birthing at home, midwives must have a deep trust in the birthing process. Yet experienced midwives and doulas have all attended births that required an unexpected cesarean.

Birth as a wild and unpredictable event

When discussing the possibility of a hospital transport with her clients, midwife Silke Akerson says, "Most births unfold really simply and without complications at home, but birth is wild, huge, and not under our control. My job is to notice if we are not in the realm of normal anymore and to access tools at the hospital that we don't have at home."

This view of birth as a feral and unpredictable event is common among midwives. "Birth is an unknown, always. Things will come up that you didn't expect. That's just the way it is!" says midwife Heather Hack. She continues, "When my daughter was young, she wanted a dog. So we got one, and after a week she said, 'I love the dog too much; we have to get rid of it. What if she dies someday?' I told her, 'This is what life is, and you take it because it's worth it. You can't guarantee that everything's going to go the way you want. There are things that are out of our control. There is no joy without sorrow.'"

When midwives can talk with their clients about birth as an event with an unforeseeable range of outcomes, they allow the possibility that anything can happen during labor. Even in a "successful" homebirth, midwives might hear a woman report that she was shocked by how intense her contractions felt or how disappointed she was that she did not feel an instant connection to her baby. For other women, labor may be longer than imagined and the pushing may feel frustrating and unproductive. In these situations, a woman may feel blindsided, regardless of how her midwife has prepared her. If midwives can acknowledge the unpredictability of birth and normalize these feelings of disappointment, women may begin to view birth as a realm outside of their control, where even the birth's location is unknown.

When a pregnant woman has difficulty visualizing her birth, her midwife can still plant seeds of reassurance by explaining that the new mother need not feel shame in the event of a surgical birth. Midwife Susan Moray tells her clients, "Your body is strong, but sometimes things don't work out the way we all hope and want them to. And it's not something you can do anything about. There's no blame; there's just circumstance."

Other midwives strive to teach that a birthing woman's determination and willpower are small factors in her birth outcome. Midwife Pamela Echeverio tells her clients that transport and cesarean "aren't always preventable. I've given up this myth that if we do everything right, we can avoid transport. There are situations that arise when mom needs to be transported, and sometimes those will end in cesarean." When a woman hears throughout her pregnancy that she is not in control of her birth outcome and that some homebirths do end in cesareans, she has the space to experience her birth with less judgment. She can more easily accept that if she has a homebirth cesarean, she did not cause it; she can see that she did everything she could to birth her baby vaginally.

Friend or foe: Talking about the hospital
Historically, the hospital has been seen as the enemy by homebirth professionals and natural birth advocates. Some birth professionals are defensive because they perceive that hospital personnel have treated them as though they are uneducated, dogmatic, and unyielding. Other midwives fear legal action because of obstetricians' hostility towards them. Ellie Legare, midwife and HBC mother, recalls her trepidation with transporting clients early in her career. She says, "It took me a while to be in a different place with that. I wanted to avoid the hospital at all costs, and now I don't feel that way at all. It's really shifted for me, and that's great."

> *Women who are afraid of the medical model tend to be drawn to classes and books with an anti-medical message. While that message is comforting because it reinforces their beliefs and feelings, they aren't learning how to overcome their fears and negotiate being in the hospital. If a pregnant woman vilifies the medical system for performing cesareans, and she herself comes to have one, she is likely to experience shock, shame, and blame because she has already seated all women who have cesareans, including herself, as a victim and a failure.*
> —PAM ENGLAND, AUTHOR AND FOUNDER OF BIRTHING FROM WITHIN, WESTERN U.S.

Commiserating over the terrible nature of the hospital environment seems like an easy avenue for building rapport with clients in the early months of care however, when this shared animosity permeates discussions of planning for a transport and cesarean, women can feel blindsided if they need to enter the very system they have demonized. During prenatal conversations, birth professionals can foster an unbiased attitude if they describe the hospital in positive and realistic terms. The midwife, specifically, plays a key role in facilitating the move to the hospital, and her attitude can greatly influence a family's experience.

> My midwife encouraged me to become so radically opposed to everything about the hospital that, in the end, the sense of failure and mortification I felt when I ended up in that dreadful place was unbearable.
> —Bronwyn (2008, 2011/HBC; South Africa)

> I need to be ever mindful of not letting my desire to "protect" my clients from a broken maternity system get in the way of giving them the real and concrete information they'll need if they end up having to navigate that system.
> —Silke Akerson, CPM, Western U.S.

Author of *Birthing from Within*, Pam England encourages homebirth professionals to describe cesarean surgery from the mother's point of view and in honest but neutral, rather than judgmental, terms:

> While it is true that some cesareans are performed unnecessarily, and that during cesarean surgery the room is brightly lit and doctors often talk about casual topics, to only describe cesareans in a negative light suggests only one possible way of experiencing cesarean: as a victim. Instead, when each part of cesarean surgery is explained in a neutral, matter-of-fact manner, she learns the reasons, often beneficial to her, behind why things are done as they are. For example, "The lights are bright so the surgeons can see what they are doing, so they do a good job for you. Sometimes when surgeons work, they talk to each other because they can't really see the woman behind the screen. Because there is a curtain blocking the parents' faces from their view, they are actually more in relation with each other than they are with you. Fortunately, surgeons are focusing on all the little but important details of the surgery. And in this zone they don't necessarily think of a cesarean

as a meaningful birth for the mother." The same kind of explanations can be given for many of the experiences common to cesarean, such as why the woman's arms are extended, why the table is narrow, why the baby is often taken to a warmer first, and so on.

In areas of the country where certified professional midwifery is illegal, or where there is friction between midwives and hospital staff, midwives struggle to support women during transport because they fear investigations and lawsuits. Consequently, the family may not receive the continuity of care that is essential for a healthy homebirth cesarean. In such cases, the birth team needs to discuss in advance the plan for caring for a woman throughout transport and cesarean, and recommend that a couple hire a birth doula to support them in the hospital.

The hostility between hospital staff and homebirth midwives has slowly eased in some regions of the United States. For example, professional midwives in Portland, Oregon, have worked extensively to build a collaborative relationship with certified nurse midwives and obstetricians in hospitals. Dr. Duncan Nielson, Chief of Women's Services at Legacy Health System, says, "The role of the hospital is to deal with people who attempt a homebirth, but only when something doesn't go the way that they want. Our mission is good health for our people and our communities. So if our mission is to support the health needs of the community, then we have to address our role in the homebirth process. That role isn't for me to attend homebirths but for me to be a safety net and resource for the people who are doing homebirths." When the skills and interventions that the hospital staff provide are valued by homebirth midwives, and midwives are viewed in turn by the hospital staff as educated and professional, these relationships can facilitate far better hospital experiences for their mutual clients.

> I approach the topic of transports with an open mind, and share with clients that I'm really comfortable going to the hospital. I'm not a midwife who has any fear or hesitation when it comes to transport. I have friends there, I feel respected, and I have a great voice in continuing to work with my clients as an advocate when we transport. But I also add that there's a question about how my moms will be treated, because I don't know who will be on staff when we go there.
>
> —MELISSA GORDON-MAGNUS, CPM, WESTERN U.S.

I have a great backup situation with a doctor who treats my women with respect and gentleness because she really trusts me. I have the privilege of not feeling hesitant if I have to transport someone, and not being afraid of how she will be treated. Transport is a continuation of the woman's birth journey.
—MARY JACKSON, RN, LM; WESTERN U.S.

Because I live in a state where midwifery is illegal, when I transport a family, I go in as a doula with a fake name. I make sure the family never says my name in the hospital.
—JENEVIVE JACOBS, CPM, MIDWESTERN U.S.

Beyond the basic hospital plan

Bryan Baisinger, DC, owner of an integrative health and wellness clinic, says, "The traumatic cesarean isn't a failure in labor; it can be a consequence of a lack of planning prenatally. Women who have unexpected cesareans often hadn't considered that they may need a surgical procedure to complete the birth process. Prenatal planning can help move a woman through what she needs to do to bring her baby onto the planet."

Legally, midwives are minimally required to complete a written hospital transport plan and explain to clients what constitutes an emergent and non-emergent transport. Beyond the basics, though, the birth team can encourage clients to tour their chosen hospital prenatally. Counselor Brooke Noli, whose words began this chapter, says, "I'm a fan of telling people prenatally that they should check out the hospital. Go, walk around, visit the café, get a doughnut or just park in the parking lot. Even that may be too much for some people, and they just don't want to—sometimes they choose homebirth because they hate hospitals."

Becoming more familiar with the hospital allows a woman and her partner to see what the environment is actually like, and imagine what it might feel like to birth there. A woman who is afraid or anxious about hospitals may find that simply walking into one on her own terms may lessen her worry and allow her to feel more confident in the event of a cesarean.

My midwife encouraged me to tour the hospital and that was one of the things that laid the groundwork for it not being so terrifying. I had already been in

that building, I knew where things were located, and I understood what their
philosophies were.
—RACHEL (2011/HBC, WESTERN U.S.)

In addition to touring the hospital, one critical piece of the prenatal transport and cesarean plan is clarifying who will accompany the family to the
hospital and remain with them throughout the birth. In many cases, HBC
mothers we interviewed were shocked to find that their midwives had no
intention of meeting them at the hospital, and they had made no alternative plans if the midwife was unable to attend the hospital birth. Women
need the birth team's continuous support when transporting and should
know the backup plan ahead of time.

To help ease the discomfort that may be present during uncomfortable
prenatal conversations, Amanda Roe, a naturopathic midwife, gives her
clients the schedule of when she will discuss a hospital transport plan and
interventions, including cesarean. This provides families with an opportunity to prepare for potentially difficult discussions. During these conversations, she asks them what they have heard about cesarean and invites them
to share their feelings, questions, or concerns. With a better understanding
of a family's uneasiness, Roe can delve deeper into addressing fears that
may impact a woman's potential cesarean birth experience.

Midwife Pamela Echeverio spends time educating clients on how she will
assess the mother's and baby's health during labor: "I think it's important
to explain to clients what we do, and that starts prenatally. For example, in
the course of labor, when we are evaluating if the baby is doing well, clients
understand what it means when we say that we are hearing heart decelerations. They have that foundation of knowledge, so when we are talking
about transport, they know the language. They need to understand that
they are part of the decision when it comes time to leave home."

Families feel overwhelmed by the choices they need to make when entering the hospital, particularly after a long and difficult labor, or after a fast
change of plans pre-labor. For a couple who has had ample opportunity to
discuss with their midwife each intervention, the shift to simply consenting to or declining procedures in the hospital is frustrating and disempowering. Silke Akerson asks her clients to think about how they can take

ownership of the situation if they transport. "We talk about how informed choice works in the hospital," she says, "and what kinds of questions you should ask to get your needs met." Akerson points out that it's possible to refuse certain interventions in the hospital, but that this "looks really different from saying no at home."

A midwife might offer to break her client's water to speed up her labor at home but will not perform this intervention without the client's clear understanding of the procedure and consent. If the woman declines, the midwife will offer alternatives or suggest postponing the decision until the woman is ready to make a choice. In a hospital, though, the physician often assumes that she will consent and may not wait for her verbal approval before initiating the procedure. If she refuses the procedure, she will need to clearly verbalize her choices, sometimes repeatedly. She may be pressured to consent nonetheless, or may be treated poorly if she declines other interventions.

> Prenatally our midwife told us what we needed to know so my husband and I could discuss what we were comfortable with and under what circumstances we would want to leave home. When we actually did need to transport, we didn't question whether we would go or not; we had a plan and we knew what to expect. It was good to have the information we needed ahead of time because we weren't thinking very clearly in the moment.
> —Heidi (2003/HBC, 2008/VBAC, 2009/RCS; Southern U.S.)

Following a mother's lead

In some situations, a midwife or doula might allow the mother to guide how much discussion she wants to have about transport and cesarean. Internationally recognized midwife and educator Mary Jackson says that for her:

> It really depends on the woman. Sometimes I have a client whose framework is such that she only wants to speak the positive. She believes that if we talk about anything negative, it will somehow draw the negative to her. I say, "I have some information about the hospital to give, are you open to hearing that?" These women will say, "No, because that's not going to happen to me." And I'll reply that most women do not expect it to happen to them, and that some women find it useful to hear logistics about what would happen if they did need to

transport. Others still don't want to hear about it. So I leave it up to the woman, and if she doesn't want to hear about the hospital, I refer her to books where she can read more about it. Other people will feel comfortable and want to hear about it, and we'll talk about transport in the depths that they want to go.

A few midwives we interviewed share transport and cesarean information only if a client asks. Midwife Jenevive Jacobs reports that she discusses transport "only in the interview. It doesn't come up again unless they ask questions."

Renowned birth expert Elizabeth Davis acknowledges that midwives should be forthcoming with information, but "the bottom line is that any woman, at any time, can investigate cesarean birth if she's curious about it. In the best of all worlds, where women are responsible for themselves and their healthcare, they don't wait for their care provider to advise them on this but go out and find the information themselves."

Barriers to prenatal discussions

While most birth professionals want their clients to be knowledgeable about all possible outcomes, and most mothers want to understand what may happen during birth, there exist multiple emotional and cultural barriers that can keep this from happening.

> *My midwife didn't do a lot that made me feel prepared about transporting to the hospital. And if someone had tried to tell me, I would have said I didn't need that information. We need midwives who aren't afraid to talk about it and who are equipped to emotionally handle it themselves, as well as a woman who is ready for it.*
> —SUE (2010/HBC, WESTERN U.S.)

With few exceptions, the mothers and partners we interviewed felt their midwives, doulas, or childbirth educators did not prepare them for their transport and cesarean. Many women felt blindsided by transport, lacked detailed information on procedures and care options, and did not have a realistic understanding of recovery and the postpartum period after a cesarean birth.

While the families expressed disappointment in how inadequately their birth teams addressed these topics, the midwives we interviewed shared that clients are often resistant to the possibility of anything less than an ideal home-birth. When the topics of transport and cesarean are raised, clients are often unwilling to consider them as a reality. If midwives agree that discussing cesarean birth with clients is critical, why is there still a lack of understanding and dialogue on both sides? What is the role of the midwife, doula, and childbirth educator in this communication breakdown?

> We talked about why we might transfer and what we would do in that case, but they never talked to me about the possibility of a cesarean. Can you imagine teaching pilots how to fly planes, but not what to do in case of a crash landing? Empowering women means giving them a complete set of tools, not treating them like children who can't handle hearing about the tough scenarios.
> —BETH (2009/HBC, WESTERN U.S.)

> My cesarean prep was absolutely not adequate. When I asked them, the midwives were willing to talk about transfer and get detailed about it, but not when it came to cesarean. They just didn't talk about it at all.
> —DANA (2012/HBC, WESTERN U.S.)

> When I wasn't practicing my childbirth exercises, my midwife scolded me by telling a story about a mom who didn't prepare enough for birth and had a long labor and cesarean. That was really the only time she ever brought up cesarean with me, which is probably why I was so caught off guard when it happened.
> —CHRISTINE (2009, 2012/HBC; NORTHEASTERN U.S.)

> I care about my midwives and I know they care about me. My heart is heavy when I think of this, but I really feel like they could have done better preparing me. We would talk about transport but never, ever cesarean. Even as I was in an ambulance with a breech baby, I thought I was going to have a vaginal birth. I feel stupid for not knowing that.
> —CAROL (2012/HBC, WESTERN U.S.)

> You don't want to scare people who are trying to have a homebirth, but it's a good idea to know things. My midwives did a great job with the idea of trans-

port. I wrote a birth plan, but it wasn't the same as being mentally prepared
for a cesarean. I don't remember talking about that at all.
—ALEXIS (2011/HBC, MIDWESTERN U.S.)

We had a total of two transport conversations that I specifically brought up.
My midwives were great about all of my questions. They said, "We are going
to try whatever we can at home, but if at any point something seems like a
danger to you or the baby, we are going to go to the hospital." They had a very
healthy view towards the hospital, where it's a tool that may need to be used.
But cesarean was never mentioned.
—BRANDY (2011/HBC, MIDWESTERN U.S.)

For a woman planning to birth out-of-hospital, choosing to consider what would happen during transport may require colossal mental and emotional shifts. To discuss the possibility of cesarean may be terribly upsetting, and may further dismantle her vision of birth. However, if midwives can explain clearly why this is important and what might happen upon arrival at the hospital, women may feel less traumatized after an HBC, resulting in healthier postpartum transitions.

Magical thinking

During prenatal visits, women may ask their birth team about cesarean, express fears, or share stories of friends who had surgical births. Some birth professionals use this opportunity to fully explore a woman's concerns, but others falsely reassure her that her fears will not materialize. Midwives, doulas, and childbirth educators who are uncomfortable discussing cesarean sometimes suggest to a "worried" or "anxious" client that she should focus on manifesting the best possible outcome: a homebirth. This dismissal of a client's apprehensions can unwittingly reinforce the practice of "magical thinking," which is the faulty notion that a person can prevent an unwanted outcome by refusing to discuss or consider it.

Throughout my care the hospital wasn't touched on that much. I was always
the person saying, "But if we have to transfer, what happens?" From my mid-
wives I kept getting the message, "That's probably not going to happen to you.
You'll be fine. Don't worry." I think they thought I was afraid, but really I wanted
to know what the procedure was at the hospital. I wish their overall attitude
wasn't so promising. They trust birth so much, and that's a good thing, but it

would have been nice if they explained what would happen during a transport and asked questions about my concerns.
—Ashley (2011/HBC, Southern U.S.)

Before I switched midwives in my third trimester, when I kept asking questions about the hospital, they told me it was "time for us to start focusing on what's going to go right and visualize what I want to create." I felt like there wasn't a real opening to talk about what I was concerned about. With my second group of midwives, they did talk to me about the possibility of transport. We wrote an alternate birth plan, but they never discussed cesarean in any detail, either. I didn't feel prepared for what was actually involved in a surgery or recovery. In terms of prenatal preparation, I've gone back and forth between "Where's the blame and the responsibility?" and "Where's the letting go?"
—Rachel (2009/HBC, Western U.S.)

Pam England says that too often when mothers ask their midwives about cesareans "they are given false assurances that 'That won't happen. You're having a homebirth.' Or, 'Think positively; don't think about it or you'll make it happen.' Should a cesarean become necessary, those messages set the stage for women to blame themselves for not thinking positively *enough*, and to wonder what they did wrong."

In retrospect, I now understand that having prenatal conversations about cesareans is not going to make them happen. Homebirthers are trying hard to negate the detrimental modern ideas of childbirth. By not letting negative thoughts into their energy field, women are attempting to keep mainstream birth culture at bay. Mothers have questions about cesarean, and I look at midwives and the natural childbirth movement as needing to understand their own responses to these questions so women aren't holding these big fears on their own.
—Rachel (2009/HBC, Western U.S.)

While midwives are often too cautious, not wanting to plant seeds of negativity by discussing unwanted outcomes, women also reported that they were unwilling to discuss homebirth cesarean for fear of manifesting this outcome. If the midwife, doula, or childbirth educator does not deconstruct this naïve magical thinking with the client in a direct and sensitive manner, the woman may never be educated about the possibility.

I felt that considering going to the hospital was bad energy, and I didn't want to jinx myself. My midwife even told me that I might want to pack a bag just in case, but I refused to do that and we ended up there anyway.
—NICOLE (2011/HBC, MIDWESTERN U.S.)

During my first pregnancy, I had all kinds of confidence. My midwives talked to me about possible outcomes but I paid no attention because I wasn't one of those uneducated moms who gets all the interventions. During my second pregnancy we explored my fears about birth and thoroughly talked about what we would do if we had to transport for a cesarean. That made all the difference.
—LIBBY (2011/HBC, 2013/VBAC TRANSPORT; MIDWESTERN U.S.)

Thinking about cesarean does not cause it to magically enter the reality field and make it more possible. There is also this idea that women will be weak and give in to cesareans if they are talked about as an option. That's disrespectful to women. For mothers who have chosen an out-of-hospital birth, they have already said that cesarean is way down on the list of birth options. So we need to eliminate this idea that talking about cesarean somehow makes it more likely to happen.
—BETH (2009/HBC, WESTERN U.S.)

I didn't want to talk about it. I was in denial and didn't give that reality too much power. I wanted to keep it at bay and think positively that I was going to have a homebirth.
—BRANDY (2011/HBC, MIDWESTERN U.S.)

Midwife Sister MorningStar focuses on making a solid plan for the care of the woman and her newborn in the case of a cesarean:

It's hard to have a baby at home. Have you looked at the stats lately? In general, the thing that all women have in common is a uterus that can be cut open to birth a baby. Living or dead, this can happen. You can't walk down the street and ask a mother how her baby was born without hearing it was cut out of her. It takes a miracle to end up with what you want during birth. So it's not for weak wishing or thinking positively. A midwife and mom have got to have a plan that includes what are you going to do if the birth doesn't happen at home. What's the plan? You've got to have a plan.

Tami Lynn Kent, a women's health physical therapist and author, adds:

> Providers are concerned about the power of suggestion and energizing something too much. They can introduce homebirth cesarean by saying, "I think we're smart enough to handle this difficult conversation." Midwives and other birth professionals can get more comfortable with having these conversations and knowing that when they bring these topics up, they are trying to give them less power over all of us.

This idea of magical thinking is common among childbirth professionals and homebirthing families. In a culture where the predominant media images of birth portray laboring women in agony and begging for pain relief, midwives, doulas, and childbirth educators often feel the need to counter with a more satisfying picture of birth. When professionals focus only on "good" results, women may not realize the value of considering a wider range of outcomes and therefore miss an opportunity to build resiliency as new mothers.

> *Magical thinking keeps fears at bay and allows women to focus instead on the positive aspects and outcomes of birth. This is so important because women need to keep some distance from all of the negative birth imagery out there. The challenge is to find the balance in staying close to the normalcy of birth while also remaining a bit open to the possibility that things may not go as hoped. I'm actually a huge fan of magical thinking, but not in the way we're talking about it here. The real magic happens when women can discover the gift or empowerment in their birth experience, no matter what that experience is, and no matter how long it takes to find it. In this context the magic is happening through the birth experience itself.*
> —Brooke Noli, counselor and certified birth doula, Western U.S.

Considering cesarean

While some pregnant women employ magical thinking, others are unable to ruminate on cesarean as a real possibility for their birth because they are too fearful to examine it closely. Midwives we interviewed reported that when they discuss transport and cesarean, women often become anxious, dismissive, or simply unable to engage in the conversation.

I didn't even read the chapter on cesarean. I thought that would not happen to me. It was definitely my worst fear. My midwives said my husband and I should go to the hospital and look around to get familiar so it wasn't too scary. But we were not about to waste our time doing that. I was really shut down about it. My midwife may have brought the hospital idea up more than once, but I didn't respond very well.

—ALICIA (2009/HBC, MIDWESTERN U.S.)

We interviewed many HBC mothers who reported, like Alicia, that while they were pregnant, they could not absorb the possibility of cesarean. Some women were hoping for a peaceful home or birth center birth, or believed that preparation and healthy choices could arm them against unwanted outcomes. How do these barriers prevent women from gaining ownership of the wide range of possibilities for their births, and how can professionals guide honest and informative discussions around cesarean birth?

I tell clients that I transport 10% of the time in labor and I have a 5–7% c-section rate. I tell them that means that they could have a c-section. I mean 7%, that's not none!

—KORI PIENOVI, CNM, WESTERN U.S.

If I sense that there is resistance to talking about cesarean, I'll preface it by speaking of the HBC Facebook group (a support forum). I know so many women in that group wish that their midwife had looked them square in the eye and said something like, "A cesarean birth isn't the most likely outcome, but it is a possible outcome, and I will still be your midwife even if I'm not the one who delivers your baby." This is something I now say to everybody, and that makes it easier to move the discussion into what a homebirth cesarean can look like.

—AMANDA ROE, NATUROPATHIC MIDWIFE, WESTERN U.S.

Midwives, doulas, and childbirth educators can observe how a woman responds when discussing childbirth—from body language such as defensive postures or lack of eye contact, to a more engaged type of listening and talking. This provides valuable insight into her internal feelings about cesareans. In response, the birth professional can ask gentle, open-ended questions to guide the conversation into a safe space for the mother: "What comes up for you when we talk about cesarean? What is scary to you about having a cesarean?" Sister MorningStar, when sensing that a client is uncomfortable with the discussion of cesarean, might ask, "What are you going to do with *you* if you have a cesarean?" This question can begin to unlock a woman's deeper feelings and worries, and then allow her to move into proactive planning, or at least open consideration of a potential cesarean.

Mother's worst nightmare

For some women, the idea of a cesarean birth is so bleak and terribly unwanted that they consider it their "worst nightmare." When this is the case, having frank discussions about cesarean is difficult, especially when women are looking ahead to birth as an already unpredictable event. MorningStar notes that if it becomes clear to her that a mother's biggest fear is cesarean, and if she says she does not want to think about it, then she "would tell her it sounds really important to talk about and ask her what we should do if we have to deal with that situation. Then we would start making a plan."

> There actually is something worse that could happen to cesarean mothers. I understand that they perceive a cesarean as the worst thing that ever happened, but I know from experience that some women don't get a live baby.
> —LIZ ROBINSON, CNM, WESTERN U.S.

Kori Pienovi asks her clients how they would feel about a cesarean. "If they say, 'that's my biggest fear,' I say really gently, 'That's not the worst that could happen. A loss is much worse.'" Pienovi encourages women to walk themselves through a scenario in which they would say, "I want a cesarean for this baby." "It's scary for them, but I want them to see where they might choose to have a cesarean in some situations." A woman might imagine that after hours of pushing with no progress, and with a baby showing signs of distress, that a cesarean could be the only solution for an otherwise dangerous situation. In this case, the mother might not only consent to the cesarean, she might actively decide that the surgery is her best choice given the circumstances. If she can realize the value of cesarean birth, at least in some situations, it can help her feel less trepidation about the potential surgery.

Sarah Buckley, MD, renowned birth expert and author of *Gentle Birth, Gentle Mothering*, says, "We don't want to say that the over 30% cesarean rate in hospitals is acceptable, because it's not. However, we also need to always consider that a cesarean is an important and sometimes life-saving operation. It's difficult to hold those two things in mind." If a mother can accept that a cesarean birth carries the potential to bring her across the threshold to motherhood with a live baby, and that this might otherwise be impossible, she may develop a more thoughtful acceptance of surgical birth. This evolving acceptance may then allow her to begin to make realistic backup plans for her birth experience.

It is also helpful for the midwife, doula, and childbirth educator to point out prenatally that women who have an HBC often feel a terrible amount of grief, despite its necessity. These feelings are valid, and important for mothers to process in order to begin healing. If the expectant woman expresses significant fear of cesarean that cannot be resolved during prenatal visits or childbirth classes, the birth team can provide her with referrals to mental health professionals who specialize in perinatal mental health, and advise her to begin the difficult work of examining her fears.

Once a woman has begun to address her concerns about a cesarean birth, she can constructively formulate a written plan in case she does need a cesarean. Plan C, found in Appendix A, outlines the many choice-points women may have during a surgical birth. Plan C can be a starting point for women to regain a sense of control and empowerment in their birth planning and postpartum care if it veers in an unwanted direction. The Plan C worksheet can guide prenatal discussions between the mother, partner, and birth team, and it is a robust tool for negotiating with the hospital staff.

How we are born matters

In addition to reframing the life-saving intention of cesarean, and adding perspective, a woman can find clues about her own internalized fears by knowing how she herself was born, and how her own mother's labor unfolded. Some midwives ask women about their own birth on the health history form in order to link it with reactions she may experience when she gives birth to her child. Mary Jackson explains the link between a woman's fears in labor and her own birth:

> The baby growing inside its mother's body perceives the mother as its outer being, with no real distinction between what the mother experiences and what the baby experiences. If the mother has a fear of the

hospital or an intervention that's about to happen, then the baby learns something about labor through that experience. Let's say the mother is in fear as she enters transition. When that baby grows up and is giving birth herself, right when she hits transition, it may trigger a memory of what was scary for her mother.

Our brain isn't able to timestamp these intrauterine memories and understand that they are from the past. If fear is coming from her own birth, then I work with the mother to differentiate that that's what was happening to her mother, and that she's working to do something really different with herself and her own baby.

This reflection on her history can provide a mother with an opportunity to deeply explore her fears or visceral reactions to pregnancy and the upcoming birth experience, and give her time to seek counseling and practice coping techniques before labor.

I can control this, right?

When women have prepared to give birth by reading books, taking classes, and eating well, it can be shocking to end up with a birth that doesn't meet their expectations. Pregnant women often seek comfort in believing that if they do the "right" things, then they will be rewarded for their efforts by having a satisfying birth, easy nursing, and a healthy baby.

This illusion of control drives humans to make better decisions, yet it also leads people to believe that they hold more power over circumstances than they actually do. For a homebirthing woman, it is often incomprehensible to accept that her willpower, educated choices, and desires are only a small component in a greater picture of how labor and birth will unfold. The baby's position, the woman's pelvic structures, and her individual cocktail of labor hormones, among countless external factors, all play a role in determining a woman and baby's unique roadmap of labor and birth. If a baby is misaligned, no matter a woman's sheer determination or her midwife's expert advice and care, that mother may still need a surgical birth. Birth professionals can discuss what the mother can do to optimize her chances of having a homebirth, such as eating well, staying fit, and reducing stress, but they can also temper their client's expectations of retaining control over the labor and birth process.

I'm a perfectionist and always believed that you can control anything as long as you do all the right things. My HBC was a huge life lesson that that's not true. You can do everything that birth expert Ina May Gaskin would ever want you to do and still end up with something different from what you wanted.
—ANN (2011/HBC, MIDWESTERN U.S.)

I skipped the chapter on cesarean because it wasn't going to happen to me. I wasn't laboring in the hospital and I wasn't going to have the cascade of medical interventions. I went to medical school, I saw videos of surgery, I attended births, and I knew what happened during a cesarean. But I had no clue about what would happen to ME if I had a cesarean.
—KORIN (2006, 2012/HBC; WESTERN U.S.)

Be wise enough to think you are not above being sent to the hospital. I look back and see I was too arrogant to consider transport as a real possibility.
—BRYANNA (2010/HBC, 2012/HBAC; WESTERN U.S.)

Midwife Amanda Roe observes that though she openly talks about HBC, "I still find it difficult to engage women in a candid conversation about all the steps involved in cesarean. The belief that 'it's not going to happen to me because I've done my research' is alive and well within the walls of my practice."

High expectations and romanticizing birth

We set the bar really high when it comes to birth by romanticizing and making it like a spiritual experience. As opposed to 'life happens' and some births are easy and some are not so easy. It's not a bad thing, but it can be a bigger crash if a woman does that.
—KAREN JACKSON FORBES, PSYCHOTHERAPIST, WESTERN U.S.

Many HBC mothers have shared that they heard very few, if any, HBC birth stories while they were pregnant. Women who plan to give birth out-of-hospital tend to seek much of their information within the natural birthing community, and that community predominantly showcases uncomplicated homebirths. "The dream of homebirth can involve singing bowls, candles, and massages," says Corrine Porterfield, a practitioner of Maya Abdominal Therapy and Maya Spiritual Healing. "Women share their amazing homebirth stories, and deep in our hearts and souls, we yearn for that experience. That strong desire makes it hard to consider other possibilities. But when you are open to many possibilities, you have a little more freedom in your experience."

> *Many women are in distress after having a cesarean when they were planning a homebirth, because they had a preconceived script of what the birth would be like. So many things are unpredictable and we need to do everything we can to make it easier for mothers.*
> —MICHEL ODENT, MD, BIRTH EXPERT AND AUTHOR, UNITED KINGDOM

Midwife Ingrid Andersson describes what she often sees with first-time parents:

> They want their perfect birth because they were raised with high expectations of themselves and they want their caregivers to help them achieve that. The result, when a woman has unrealistic goals for herself, her partner, and her midwives, is that she will be disappointed by her birth experience. Our culture has gotten away with an unbalanced view of birth, because we don't live that close to the marrow of life. Our lives are distorted in that people should always look good, never be dirty, never poop in public. That's just not real life.

Generations ago, young women on the verge of becoming mothers had already seen other women in their family give birth, and they understood that labor is arduous, painful, and can result in less than ideal outcomes. In first-world countries, women today are unlikely to witness birth first hand, and may have only viewed highly edited, unrealistic birth footage, and used those images to calibrate their expectations of how their own birth will proceed.

> *There is something about the first experience of going through the birth door, it's just hard to comprehend what's about to happen. First-time moms often are not aware of the realities of birth as most have never witnessed birth before they give birth themselves. Talking about different birth outcomes actually gives women more skills to handle their own labor.*
> —TAMI LYNN KENT, WOMEN'S HEALTH PHYSICAL THERAPIST AND AUTHOR, WESTERN U.S.

Even experienced mothers can be shocked by the reality of a homebirth cesarean. A woman who already gave birth vaginally may have very little reason to consider the possibility of a cesarean—after all, her body has pushed babies out before and will likely do so again. She may also be thinking, "This is my last baby. I want this one to be perfect!" In building her high expectation that this upcoming birth will trump the others in its ease, speed, and beauty, there is bound to be some level of disappointment and grief, particularly when confronted by an HBC.

The role of childbirth educators
In addition to midwives and doulas helping mothers prepare for the possibility of cesarean, childbirth educators play a pivotal role in addressing this potential outcome in their classes. Pam England says:

> Most homebirthers are holding onto a story that the hospital is a bad place. A child talks like that: in absolutes and black and white. The hospital is a medical building and the people in it are ordinary people. It's important for a homebirth mom to know ahead of time that if she goes to the hospital during labor, then in all likelihood she needs to be there. Childbirth classes are a great place to bring this up, because it can be a little easier to discuss these interventions in a group setting. If it's part of a class, then maybe moms will pay attention more and not feel like it's directed at them.

Jesse Remer, childbirth educator and doula, believes that all pregnant women need to have a conversation about induction, epidural, and cesarean. She tells homebirth families that they are:

> still going to have to open this door and look at it even though they are planning an out-of-hospital birth. Sometimes women are making a choice to have birth out of the hospital because they are against these things. Even if they are opposed to an epidural, they still need to have the conversation about it. I also share with families that when unexpected interventions happen, I often hear women say, "That's the one thing I didn't want to have happen." Often that "one thing" has never been talked about. Talking about this means women can at least try it on and identify their highest intention if they had to have the intervention. I ask them when they build a birth plan, what's the feeling they

want to generate in their birth? If a woman says "peace," we figure out how she can generate peace if she has a cesarean.

Julia, an HBC mother who took one of Remer's childbirth classes, recalls:

> The other people were planning hospital births, so Jesse took me aside and said, "You should talk to your midwife about the possibility of transport, what would happen, and how would you want that to go." At the time, I felt so confident about my birth that I blew it off a little, but I did take it seriously enough that I talked with my midwife. After my birth, I felt really glad that Jesse did say something. I wish I had seen c-section as a real possibility. I was in that mindset that c-sections happened to women who weren't prepared and somehow I was. At the end of the day I felt really grateful to Jesse because if she hadn't said anything I wouldn't have discussed transfer at all with my midwives.

These prenatal discussions, particularly in a group environment, can allow women to face their fears, which helps them to be better equipped to deal with a transport and cesarean. Comparing Julia's experience with other HBC mothers' prenatal education experience, we can see how helpful Remer's approach can be.

> *My childbirth class covered transport but skirted around cesarean. It was like a taboo subject. They didn't want to talk to us about cesarean, because they didn't want us to be in a negative state of mind where we could actually make transport and cesarean a reality.*
> —LUISA (2011/HBC, WESTERN U.S.)

> *In my meditative childbirth class, the word cesarean never came up.*
> —CHRISTINE (2009, 2012/HBC; NORTHEASTERN U.S.)

> *We did cover transfer and cesarean in our class but very lightly. Honestly, I was so freaked out by the idea that I was in denial it was a possibility. I remember crying during the talk on cesarean.*
> —DANA (2012/HBC, WESTERN U.S.)

We took a class at our birth center and they didn't cover anything about trans-
ports. It was all roses, gumdrops, and the fluffy birth stuff. I met someone in
the class who had a cesarean with her first. She stopped attending the classes
because she was so upset that they hadn't even bothered to bring up cesarean
as a possibility. Cesarean happens all the time; it's part of birth.
—MAUREEN (2009/HBC, 2012/HBAC; WESTERN U.S.)

Just as midwives should address transport and cesarean options in their prenatal care, childbirth educators can learn to incorporate these crucial topics. Tina
Lilly, cofounder of a childbirth education business, interviewed with us before
she became part of the HBC online community. In her interview she said that:

Transport and cesarean fall into a discussion around birth fears. We
focus very minimally on these topics. While I find it is useful to have
couples informed about how to prepare if they need to make a hospital
decision, I also feel like I don't want to make this a very big part of
childbirth preparation. Where does the mother want to put her intention? I don't want to have a class that focuses on all the stuff that goes
wrong. Rather, I want to focus a lot more on the positive aspects of
birth and how they can actually make that happen.

Months later, after listening to HBC mothers talk about how unprepared
they were for their HBCs, Lilly's focus changed.

I am now much more upfront about the possibilities birth entails, and
I understand it's simply disempowering not to talk about all that can
happen. We are now including cesarean birth as a conversation topic
for our mostly homebirth clientele.

We have moved away from a "natural" emphasis toward a focus on
the "primal" energy of birth. A focus on "natural" birth reinforces the
idea that only vaginal, unmedicated births are real births. This is not
what we want for the couples who take our class. Approaching birth as
primal, versus natural, stretches the concept of birth to include all possible ways of bringing a child into the world, without discarding any of
the natural aspects of childbirth. We believe that it better captures the
essence of birth, which is to bring a baby into the world, and to have
mother and baby survive.

In Tina's classes, we did an exercise where everyone picked a card out of a basket of labor problems. The card we got was everything that wound up happening in my birth: long labor, transfer, emergency cesarean. I started panicking about it after class, but because of this exercise, I knew a little of what to expect. If we hadn't gotten the crappiest card in class, I wouldn't have been able to think about it prenatally.
—ALISSA (2011/HBC, WESTERN U.S.)

Scarlett Lynsky, cofounder of a childbirth preparation business, describes one full class of their education series that is focused on interventions: "Because we have a mix of hospital and homebirth families, we make it clear that the homebirthers should also be thinking about interventions and cesarean because of the real possibility of transport. Almost everyone in my classes wants to avoid cesarean, but if a mom needs one and is able to take time along the way to make conscious choices, it can feel better in the end, even if it is a radical departure from what her goal is."

My childbirth class with Scarlett saved the day. Most of the people were homebirthers, but they really taught us about cesarean and how to make it as close to natural as you can. At the time, I didn't want to hear it, but because we had those classes, my experience was so much better. We had time to learn and process it. That is invaluable for anyone giving birth.
—CARRIE (2011/HBC, WESTERN U.S.)

What mothers want

What are some ways to bring prenatal conversations to an honest middle ground so women can feel as prepared as possible for an out-of-hospital birth and a cesarean? To answer this question, it can be helpful to reflect on the experiences of women who have had a homebirth cesarean and went on to give birth again. The birth warriors we interviewed shared that they went into their next pregnancy armed with a very clear idea of how they wanted to talk about transport and cesarean. These mothers who have walked through the fire of surgical birth knew what they needed from their birth teams to feel safe, supported, and prepared for any outcome. (See Chapter 12 for more information on subsequent pregnancies after an HBC.)

During my first pregnancy, the most we ever talked about transport was about where to go. With my second, we talked about it a lot with our birth team:

how I was feeling, emotional stuff around transport and cesarean, how our midwives felt about it. And we had a plan for every scenario.
—KORIN (2006, 2012/HBC; WESTERN U.S.)

Because we spent so much time talking about my fears and concerns, and what was important to me, my midwives knew what I wanted when I was too distressed to verbalize it. They were able to advocate for me when I couldn't.
—TARA (1999/VAGINAL HOSPITAL BIRTH, 2006/CS, 2008, 2010/HBC; WESTERN U.S.)

These women were careful to hire midwives and doulas who understood their needs for emotional support, information, and clear communication throughout their care. Additionally, they had clarity around their own boundaries for birth—how long they wanted to labor at home before considering transport, tuning into their intuition to make decisions, and choosing who should be present at the birth.

Planning for postpartum support
During the course of prenatal care, one of the most important jobs of midwives, doulas, and childbirth educators is to prepare clients not only for the process of giving birth, but also for what to expect in the postpartum period. Many HBC women felt they were not informed by their birth team that their healing would be compounded by the additional challenges of recovery from a surgical birth. Once a mother and her partner or support person have clearer expectations about physical and emotional healing after an HBC, the midwife and doula can address their own roles postpartum, guide the family to rally the support they will need, and show them where to seek additional help. Sister MorningStar says that as a mother "deals with reality unfolding, where is her physical, emotional, spiritual, and cultural support? That system that she wants to rely on in her postpartum time, has it worked in the past? A mother has to be mothered to mother her baby."

Realistic discussions about healing from a cesarean
If this is her first baby, a pregnant woman may have no idea what the day-to-day care for a newborn involves or how much time nourishing a baby will take. She may not even have a clear picture of what the healing process from a vaginal birth looks like, or a full understanding of the ways a cesarean birth complicates recovery, both from a physical and an emotional standpoint.

The birth team can explain both the normal flow of a postpartum day at home with a newborn and the specific ways that recovering from major abdominal surgery can make daily tasks more difficult. During a home visit, a doula might show a family how keeping diaper-changing supplies near the bed can make this task faster at night, promoting more sleep for the new mother and her partner. She might also explain that if the woman has a cesarean, her partner will need to do all the diaper changes, since leaning, crouching, and lifting the baby will be painful, and sometimes impossible, in the early weeks. This information can help families begin to deconstruct their expectations of a quick and easy recovery.

Midwives, doulas, and childbirth educators can speak candidly with pregnant women and partners about what it feels like to heal from a cesarean, and describe some common challenges and emotions the mother and her partner might experience. (See Appendix B, Caring for the HBC Mother.) A childbirth educator might describe the juxtaposition of holding gratitude for a healthy baby while mourning the loss of a homebirth. She might also share that it is common for the partner to feel less grief over this loss, and that this difference in perspective can yield tension between the couple. Through sharing postpartum scenarios and challenges, the new family can begin to envision why compassionate support will be needed after birth.

> Prenatally, we'll teach the mother to build layers of support in her life, and how to find and receive support around her. Often, the women who tend to do it all themselves don't know how to let that support in.
> —MARY JACKSON, RN, LM; WESTERN U.S.

Clarifying the birth team's role
The care a midwife provides is intensive around the time of the birth, and the mother can feel that her midwife has seemingly forgotten about her as her care tapers off in the weeks following birth. During prenatal conversations about postpartum support, the midwife can explain what her own role will be after the birth and how the amount of care she provides will decrease over time. It can also be helpful to remind women prenatally that this diminishing care from the birth team is normal for all clients, regardless of how the mother gives birth, and suggest ways to ease that transition with help from friends and family. (For postpartum support planning, see Appendix A, Plan C.)

The needs of a recovering HBC mother are vast, so each member of the birth team can explain their anticipated schedule of visits, how that time will be used, and what the scope of care will look like. The midwife or doula may share that she will be glad to offer extra home visits in the first week after the new mother arrives home from the hospital. The birth team can explain that they will take turns calling the new mother on a set daily schedule for the first few weeks, or longer if needed. This gives the mother ample opportunity to ask questions without feeling like she is bothering her midwives, allows her to stay connected to her birth team, and can help the birth team assess her wellbeing inbetween visits. If the midwife is planning to leave town, or foresees a heavy client-care load during the postpartum time, she can explain that the assistant or backup midwife will be fully available to provide support.

The midwife needs to clearly convey that her role is to provide healthcare to the mother and baby, and emotional support for the mother. If a new family's needs extend beyond her scope of training, she must communicate that she will make referrals as needed for specialized care she cannot provide, such as for chiropractors, mental health professionals, and lactation consultants.

> My job is to serve women, and part of that service is to ensure they understand how my role changes after birth. If a mom is having breastfeeding issues, I recommend a lactation professional. If she is experiencing depression or anxiety symptoms, I encourage her to seek mental health support. And if she needs extra care and love after a difficult birth, I ensure that she has trusted friends and family she can turn to.
> —JOCELYN REID, CNM, WESTERN U.S.

Helping the mother build her support network

The doula or midwife can explain the ways in which a new mother will need help from those around her. With parents who already have children, the doula may spend time brainstorming care arrangements for siblings, and ways the mother can rally dependable support from friends or family when her partner returns to work. Parents can often imagine needing assistance with chores, laundry, and caring for older children, but they may not consider gathering support for their own emotional and spiritual wellbeing after a difficult or traumatic birth. The birth team is critical in helping the family identify people who will care for and nurture the mother so that she is free to rest, heal, and feed her newborn.

Midwife and President of Birthingway College of Midwifery, Holly Scholles notes that in the traditional Mennonite community she serves, the support for a new family is extensive: "Every other night for the first two weeks, they receive a full evening meal provided by a different family. If she had a cesarean or complications, then they receive an extra week of meals. If the family has other children, then a woman from the church comes during the day to help out with childcare and housework." This level of care from the community provides the mother with not just food, but connection to others when she may need it the very most.

In addition to gaining support from the broader community of family, friends, or church members, the birth team can describe to the partner what he can do to support the mother in the early weeks after birth. The midwife might explain that if a woman has a cesarean, she will need continuous support at home for the first few weeks and that she will be recovering in bed, resting, and feeding her baby. She may have a strong need for privacy in the early days at home and will not be able to entertain guests. She might need her partner to help her remember when to take pain medications or help clean her incision if it becomes infected. The new mother might also need reassurance from her partner that someone is caring for other children, cleaning the house, and paying the bills.

The birth team can enlist the partner in monitoring the new mother's moods and wellbeing, beginning by describing common emotions she might experience after an HBC, and perhaps giving written instructions on when to check in with the team. If the new mother is single or has a partner who is unable to accomodate for her physical and emotional needs, the midwife or doula can recommend that she seek support from a family member, friend, or postpartum doula.

> *Prenatally, midwives want to be identifying the strengths in the mother's communities and families, and helping them foster those connections when thinking about their postpartum plans. Our job is assisting them in nourishing their lives and their support systems.*
> —Silke Akerson, CPM, Western U.S.

Sharing resources prenatally

Finally, the midwife, doula, or childbirth educator can give the mother a list of resources that contains trusted local counselors, therapists, and social workers, new mothers' groups, support hotlines, and physical care resources that the mother can access after birth. (See Appendix C, Resources for HBC Mothers and Families.) This resource list can also contain information for cesarean support groups such as the Homebirth Cesarean Facebook group or the Homebirth Cesarean website (www.HomeBirth-Cesarean.com) and International Cesarean Awareness Network (ICAN). Birth professionals may choose to advise their clients to initiate contact with these resources prenatally to gain a better understanding of the services they provide.

> I make sure that all my clients understand that I am an ongoing resource for them if they need referrals. Prenatally, I talk about postpartum mood disorders with all my clients to normalize that experience and help them know that I am a safe person to bring these concerns to. Long before a person is going to use a resource I leave with them, they need help recognizing their potential need for that help. I like to gently support people in coming to that realization.
> —CHRISTY HALL, CERTIFIED DOULA, WESTERN U.S.

Respecting birth and validating cesarean

When homebirth women have a surgical birth, they often experience overwhelming feelings of isolation, shame, and depression. These emotions can be further compounded if others judge or dismiss their birth experience. A newly postpartum woman might hear from family or friends that she was foolish to want a homebirth or that she was selfish for valuing her own experience over her child's safety. Her partner may not understand why she is deeply traumatized when both she and baby are now "safe." Prenatally, midwives, doulas, and childbirth educators have immense power in validating all birth outcomes, whether vaginal or cesarean.

Midwife Ellie Legare says that "from the start of care, I set it up like the hospital is not the enemy. It's not a failure if we have to go there; it's just a change of plans. You make the best decision you can, in the moment, with the information you have, to make sure that mom and baby are okay. I don't consider it a failure." If midwives can reasonably discuss transport and cesarean as a necessary change of plans and a valid way to give birth, then that removes some of the stigma for mothers and families who otherwise might feel marginalized by their HBC.

> *There are a lot of expectations and myths around natural birth that we need to clear up. The natural birth movement holds this fantasy that if a mom does everything right, she will get the birth she wants, which will prove something about her abilities, and about her as a person. This sets women up for shame because they already have expectations that communicate something about their worthiness.*
>
> *It would help if we didn't set birth expectations so high in the first place. Even saying yes to becoming a mother means you are going to meet all your inadequacies and all the places you feel vulnerable. Women don't need additional pressure about how they birth on top of that. The only thing women should strive for is to be unconditionally loving with themselves and to call in whatever they need to heal for the journey of birth and mothering.*
> —TAMI LYNN KENT, WOMEN'S HEALTH PHYSICAL THERAPIST AND AUTHOR, WESTERN U.S.

> *I understand the intentions behind the messages from the natural childbirth community. I wholeheartedly agree with their beliefs in a woman's ability to birth her baby. I don't believe for a second that birth or women are broken or that most women need the intervention of a hospital or a surgeon.*
>
> *I propose we as natural childbirth advocates respect birth. Let's respect that birth usually goes as planned with little or no intervention. Let's respect that women have adapted to giving birth successfully most of the time. Let's respect that sometimes birth doesn't go as planned. Let's respect mothers' birth stories without judging or shaming.*
> —CARA (2005, 2007/HB, 2008/HBC; WESTERN U.S.)

> *Unless we are willing to welcome cesarean into the family of "acceptable and valid" birth outcomes, we cannot have safe and effective homebirth. What we will have instead are women who feel shame and depression for having a cesarean, or who risk feelings far worse for not having one when it was needed. I was the most prepared woman ever because of my studies. That is why it kills me that women who have cesareans are portrayed as ignorant or having been taken advantage of in some way. It makes me so angry. There was nothing I could have done to prevent my cesarean.*
> —BETH (2009/HBC, WESTERN U.S.)

In addition to midwives reframing the conversation around homebirth cesarean, natural childbirth advocates can change the dialogue around birth. Instead of perpetuating the polarization of homebirth versus hospital birth, or natural birth versus cesarean birth, we can all generate a higher understanding of the appropriate use of different birth settings and choices. As Pam England says, "Can we have enough compassion to consider lots of possibilities, some of them maybe out of our control?" When we can openly present a full spectrum of births as a valid way to give birth, from a homebirth to a cesarean, mothers will find deeper satisfaction in their experiences.

Birth Professionals' Quick Guide to Prenatal Preparation

- Reinforce with clients the idea of birth as an unscripted event with a large spectrum of possible outcomes, and that all births are valid and an initiation into motherhood.

- Speak about transport, the hospital, and cesarean birth in honest, realistic, and neutral terms.

- Advise clients to take a tour of their chosen hospital to build familiarity.

- Encourage women and their partners to examine their feelings about cesarean birth rather than to employ magical thinking. Make referrals for metal health professionals if the woman remains fearful or unwilling to consider cesarean birth as a possibility.

- Assist women in developing their Plan C.

- Recommend that couples take childbirth classes that openly discuss hospital interventions, including cesarean birth.

- Discuss the cesarean birth recovery process, explain the postpartum role of the birth team, help the mother identify her support network, and offer her written resources prenatally.

Mother Love in Three Voices

WRITTEN BY: SUE BURNS, RACHAEL COOK, AND SILKE AKERSON

This birth story is written by Sue, with her partner Rachael's additions in italics. Sue and Rachael's midwife, Silke, read their story and her heartfelt response is also included. To continue the conversation, Sue's response to Silke concludes the story.

Sue: We chose our midwife because I knew that our lives were similar enough that it would be wonderful to share such an intimate thing with her. She was completely hands-off because she trusted women's bodies. She believed that birth is natural, and she was also comforting and straightforward.

I had 10 lunar months of a blissful pregnancy with excellent health and very little preparation for a hospital transport—not nearly enough education, no tour, no bag packed. My contractions started off quiet and short. I could talk through them and didn't tell Rachael, my partner of 10 years, for an hour or two as I wanted to be sure I was really in labor. And when I did tell her, we got excited! So excited that we couldn't sleep until 2 in the morning. At 4 a.m. I woke up to a POP and I knew that when I stood up, my amniotic fluid would spill out over our brand new floors. I went to the bathroom to look for blood, saw none, and woke Rachael with the news that OOOOOOHHHHHH!! the contractions were getting stronger now.

We called our midwife Silke and she came over to set up the tub. I was fearless. I trusted my body completely. I trusted the process of birth like a good feminist should.

I labored with endurance. I battled the pain and exhaustion with magic and spirit and laughter. I had a good time. I paced from one doorframe to another, leaning in for a contraction while my partner or midwife pressed on my sacrum. I vocalized. I tried to avoid the phone calls from my sister and mother, who wished I was at the hospital. I remember the sun rising twice in one day. It did not occur to me that so much time was passing. Then, on the third morning, seeing my midwife's hand shaking, I thought, "Oh no, she must be hungry or tired!" And then I realized I was failing.

I had tried so hard, and I failed. I truly believed that it was my feminist right to birth naturally, at home, in the tub, with my candles burning, with my walls around us, actualizing my careful choices. I had spent my whole life believing that I would birth a child in this way.

I knew that laboring at home was best, that birthing at home was safest, that hospital births make way for sometimes inescapable interventions, but after over 48 hours of labor with my water broken, Silke suggested we transport. I believed I was strong enough to reject that cascade of sterile, clinical, and surgical. I still had hopes of delivering vaginally, and so we left home.

Sitting in the car, 6 centimeters dilated, exhausted, dehydrated, and hungry is almost the worst part of this story. I said I hated the ride to the hospital because the road was bumpy, but the truth was that my dream was dying and I was wholly unprepared to go forward into this unchartered territory.

Rachael: The decision to transport was, after all the time Sue spent laboring, an easy decision, but such a sad choice to have to make. I knew that it was breaking Sue's heart and that broke my heart. In the movies, the couple has a bag packed and they are ready to go when their moment strikes. We had no such bag and no such moment. When we made the decision, I had nothing prepared and no plan. But, ultimately, favorite undies and a toothbrush matter much less than the fact that your hopes and dreams are being crushed. I always felt like transporting would be the "wrong" thing to do. The hospital is such an unnatural place and our whole point was to follow this course as naturally as possible.

Sue: If I had toured the hospital, met the nurses and doctors, researched hospital and surgical births AT ALL, maybe, just maybe I could have integrated my experience better. If I had opened up to the possibility that this birth was out of my control, then I could have known what drugs they were going to give me and brought homeopathics to heal. I could have entered the hospital more calmly, feeling that my needs for skin-to-skin, vaginal swabbing, and delayed cord cutting would be spoken. If I had planned for it, if I had even thought for one second that transporting was a possibility, I could have saved myself from feeling like a failure.

The hospital nurse midwife on duty said "cesarean" immediately. And there it was, my failure. I resisted an immediate cesarean and was instead hooked up to an IV and given fluids and antibiotics. Then Pitocin, an epidural, and finally after hours of pushing, I gave up. I gave in to my failure and said, "I want to meet my baby and I can't push anymore."

Prenatally, my midwife had skillfully prepared me for many of the interventions that might happen in the hospital, but not cesarean. I asked to meet the surgeon and by some karmic gift I felt intimately connected to him. I knew he could be the first person to touch my baby. I suddenly had permission to go on. If it was another person that I couldn't viscerally or spiritually connect with, then I would have had more soul loss. I wasn't going to let someone cut me open and take my baby out if I didn't love them. It's not that I would have chosen death, but that connection with this man made the cesarean less of a loss for me.

On the operating table, after 72 hours of labor, no food or sleep, dehydrated, and drugged, I hallucinated the doctor gently cutting me open and lifting my daughter out. She was ghostly white and wore a quizzical expression. I exclaimed, "It's a girl!" and Rachael looked very worried. I turned back to the light and the whole scene replayed itself, this time for real. And this time she was pink.

When my lips first touched my daughter's cheek, quieting her cries, I was initiated into a vast and deep legacy of mother love. I understood how I was loved, how endlessly I would love from then on, and how indeed, the world was held together by love. Mother love. This insight didn't keep me from feeling like a failure, but it did drive me to heal.

The days after my birth were the hardest of my life. Not panic, exactly, but filled instead with shame and survival. Having a newborn was hard. Having an identity crisis because I was a homebirther who didn't birth at home? Crushingly hard. Because I got the "at least your baby is healthy" comment so often, so quickly, I immediately sequestered myself. I did not want to hear that bullshit line. I felt invalidated. I did not want to look anyone in the face. I did not want anyone to see my shell-shocked, terrorized eyes and say, "But you are alive!" I wanted and needed someone to say, "You are incredible. You are so strong. You are a mother. You obviously have out-of-this-world endurance and resilience!" Or better yet, "Yes, it hurts. It sucks you didn't get to birth at home. I'm here for you."

No one was going to say those things because they didn't know how to handle my grief. As a culture, we don't do grief. Surgical birth is looked down on by the homebirth world. It's one of the most basic tenets of the natural birth community—either you were lazy or you were emotionally blocked or you WOULD have had a beautiful, orgasmic homebirth in the tub. I obviously wasn't lazy. And I wasn't emotionally blocked, but I didn't get my homebirth.

Rachael: When we came home from the hospital, I felt immense relief and freedom. At the same time, my entire world came crashing down. Everything I had expected from our birth experience, except for our wonderful, healthy baby, had been shattered. Now I had to, with no sleep for five days, somehow stare this right in the face and take care of our newborn child. While trying to balance the care of myself with the care of a newborn, I was failing at protecting Sue in the ways that she needed. What I didn't realize was that the intensity that I was feeling was only a fraction of what was happening for Sue. I was so incredibly unprepared for coming home, much more so than actually being in the hospital. I did not know how to support Sue and meet my own needs for sleep and nutrition. Finding this balance might have been easier if the possibility of transport and cesarean aftercare had been explored more, either with our midwife or in our birthing class.

Sue: I had to stay in my self-imposed prison until 1) I could handle my own grief, 2) I didn't need someone else to say the right thing, and 3) I could deconstruct the kind of positive thinking that had led me there. I honestly believed because I wanted a homebirth, I could have it. There's entitlement there. My emotional world had cracked open. I was raw and vulnerable. I had anxiety and no one understood.

I came out slowly. I came out guarded. I eventually accepted my cesarean. I had prepared in the best way I knew possible, I tried for a beautiful homebirth, and I ended up being transported and having a c-section.

I finally was able to say those things to myself. I labored at home for a ridiculously long time. I endured. I had stamina and an unbelievably high pain tolerance. And then I did the thing I most didn't want to do: I went to the hospital. I was brave enough to let someone cut me open and have major abdominal surgery AWAKE! so that I could be her mother. I am a warrior.

Silke, Sue's midwife responds:
When I read Sue and Rachael's birth story, I felt this big rush of sadness and shame that surprised me. They are my neighbors and friends, and we have talked in great depth about their birth experience over the years. Yet I still feel deep sadness and regret about all they have been through and about my inability to prepare them for their birth experience. In some way I still believe that I should have been able to "protect" them from having a cesarean.

I also felt a more personal sadness about the ways that my care doesn't show up in their story. The conversations that we did have about transport, the many things that we tried over days of labor to shift the baby's position and the contraction pattern, the 19 hours of labor support in the hospital after transport, the extra postpartum visits in the hospital and at home, the referrals made for physical, emotional, and spiritual healing—are all dwarfed by the very solitary experiences of exhaustion, disappointment, and trauma.

This makes sense to me, but it leaves me with big open questions. Is it possible for me to prepare clients for the experience of transport and cesarean in a way that will make it less traumatic? Is there a way I can more fully show up so a client doesn't feel so alone, or is there something about birth/surgery/trauma that a person can only go through alone?

At the same time, I also feel great happiness and gratitude when I reflect on Sue and Rachael's birth experience from my own vantage point. What I remember is their incredible strength, creativity, humor, and resilience. I remember them making the hospital room their own, filling it with their people and jokes and possessions. I remember them taking their time to understand each and every decision and asking for space when they needed it. I remember Sue interviewing both the anesthesiologist and the surgeon in order to know who they were, to establish a sense of relationship with the people who were going to remove her sensation, cut open her body, and bring her baby into the world. I remember her powerful decision-making. I remember her brilliance in restoring her boundaries at home after an experience of so many unknown people in her intimate birthing space. I remember their willingness to share this experience with me and their honesty about what I could have done differently to ease their journey.

One of the things that is clear to me from working with Sue and other HBC moms is that I need to be open to learning and changing my care in response to their experiences. And at the same time, I MUST remember that I am just one person and cannot be responsible for all of the factors beyond my care. No matter how hard I work and no matter how attentive and responsive I am, my care cannot compensate for what is broken in the hospital system or for what is lacking in our communities and cultures. I need to give my clients information and support in navigating these systems, but I can't magic away the problems by not talking about them. My clients' journeys are not mine.

Sue responds:
Such a deep hole, the loss of my homebirth. I have some guilt for bringing Silke down with me, and for not seeing or appreciating her care in my story. Silke was amazing. She labored alongside me for all 70 hours of the ordeal. She was clever, patient, knowledgeable, and wise. She not only gave me space but HELD SPACE for the birth I wanted to have. She came to the hospital and acted as my greatest support. She visited me every day in the hospital. She visited me at least weekly for months and was so patient and empathic to my grief. She gave me the single greatest healing tool—story-telling to my baby.

Here's the thing: Even with excellent preparation for a homebirth in all ways—physical, intellectual, spiritual, and emotional, even with positive thinking, even with an amazing midwife, even with a working knowledge of hospital births, interventions, and c-sections, even with a family-centered surgical birth with immediate skin-to-skin delayed cord clamping, and vaginal swabs for good gut colonization, even with heaps of therapy and support afterwards, a homebirth cesarean still sucks. Losing a homebirth is a life-changing grief.

Chapter 3

Leaving and not coming back

I knew that this baby was going to die if we didn't immediately transport. I couldn't connect with him at all. During the fast car ride to the hospital, I could feel a body part coming out, and I was holding my friend's hand, trying not to push. When we got to the emergency room, the doctors were there waiting for me with the operating room already prepped. They brought me to labor and delivery, and I was left all alone since my midwife refused to transport with me.

I began to leave my body, and I was looking down at myself from above. It was the worst experience of my life. The nurses and doctors were panicking because I came in with what we now know was an arm in my vagina.

In the operating room I was negotiating for some things, but I was in such shock and was throwing up the whole time. Suddenly, my baby was out and nobody said a word to me. I kept asking if he was okay, but nobody would answer me. He didn't even cry. It felt like he was born dead. I told my husband to go with the baby as they wheeled him to the NICU.

I didn't get to see or hold him. I actually didn't really believe that I had a baby. I thought it was all a sick joke. I remember thinking, "I don't really have a baby, maybe this is all a dream—maybe I wasn't even pregnant." I totally lost it. It was like I left my body and I couldn't get back.
—ELLIE (2006/HBC, 2010/HBAC; WESTERN U.S.)

Humans are beautifully adapted to survive in a stunning variety of life-threatening situations, yet the mental and emotional fallout that results from these intense and terrifying experiences can cause both immediate and long-term negative consequences. When experiencing a traumatic HBC, the birthing woman's nervous system interprets this sudden change of plans as an assault not just to her physical body but to her whole being, including her emotional and mental safety.

In this chapter, we explain how the nervous system responds in the face of stressful and traumatic events, and how these responses apply to women experiencing an HBC. We also delve into the fallout after trauma and ways that midwives, doulas, and partners can help facilitate a positive transition from a homebirth to a cesarean.

The nervous system

A complex relationship exists among a woman's brain, bodily sensations, and the emotions resulting from an HBC. To understand how the brain and body work together, it can be helpful to review the basic geography of the human nervous system.

The nervous system is composed of an intricate web of nerves that radiate throughout the body, the spinal cord, and the brain. The brain itself is made up of three major sections, plus the limbic system:

1)		The *brainstem* is the most primitive part of the brain and is common to all animals. It relays sensory information such as heat, touch, pressure, and pain. The autonomic nervous system is contained within the lower brainstem and spinal cord, and it serves as the control center for largely involuntary functions of the organs and glands, such as breathing and heart function, body temperature regulation, involuntary muscle movement, digestion, perspiration, sexual arousal, and urination. The autonomic nervous system is further divided into two subsystems:
	i)	The *sympathetic nervous system* quickly mobilizes responses, including immediate hormone release, prompting the fight-or-flight response.
	ii)	The *parasympathetic nervous system* more slowly activates the dampening of alarm responses, which is often described as "rest and digest" or "feed and breed," and it is responsible for the freeze response.
2)		The *cerebellum* coordinates voluntary muscle movement, posture, and balance.

3)	The *cerebrum* is divided into the right and left hemispheres, and it is the most recently evolved part of the brain. These hemispheres house different lobes that are responsible for the infinitely complex maze of functions involved in communication, memory, learning, problem-solving, judgment, emotions, movement, and other tasks that ensure that the owner of the brain survives and thrives.
4)	The *limbic system* lines the lower portion of the cerebrum. This system includes complex structures such as the amygdala and the hippocampus, which are largely responsible for human emotion, behavior, social interaction, sense of smell, and memory formation.

The stress response: Fight-or-flight

When a person first perceives acute danger or encounters a stressful situation, the limbic system activates key areas in the brain to initiate the immediate release of stress hormones called catecholamines, and epinephrine, a neurotransmitter. These chemical signals trigger activity, on behalf of the sympathetic nervous system, throughout the entire body—from the eyes down to the tiny capillaries of the toes. The uterus is situated along the route of the sympathetic nervous system and is also activated during a stress response.

Imagine, in the middle of the night, a woman waking to the sound of a shattering window in her home. She experiences a dramatic set of reactions that prepare her body to deal with the possible intruder:

- Her heart and respiratory rates increase to oxygenate her muscles so she can fight or flee the aggressor.

- Blood sugar surges, released by her liver, to give her quick access to stored energy.

- Her digestion and immune systems cease functioning, allowing her to focus on the threat to her safety.

- Her hands and feet become cold as blood is shunted to her vital organs and large muscles, which are tense and ready for action.

- Cold sweat breaks out at her brow, groin, and armpits, preventing her body from overheating in the anticipated struggle.

- Her tense body shakes, her mouth is dry, and she sees through tunnel vision that a shadowy figure is emerging from the doorway.

This *fight-or-flight* stress response is a biological adaptation to increase the odds of survival in periods of immediate danger, and it allows humans, along with reptiles and non-human mammals, to instantly access the physiological resources that would otherwise take longer to coordinate and mobilize. For the woman in the intruder scenario, her autonomic nervous system's ability to kick in and rally her body's resources allows her to defend herself against or flee from the intruder. In this case, she jumps out of bed and escapes to a neighbor's house.

Once she is safe in the home of her neighbor and she has the ability to call the police, she will notice her sheer exhaustion and the gradual resumption of normal body functions. She might feel her empty stomach rumbling and nibble on toast as she replays the events of the night over and over in her mind, recalling minute new details. As the stress hormones ebb, giving way to the sympathetic nervous system's rest and digest response, the woman can once again look to her day ahead and the task of securing her home against further invasion.

Tend and befriend

Early studies on the stress response were first conducted on animals, and then on human males, since women's fluctuating hormone levels made it more difficult for scientists to accurately measure and assess outcomes. In recent years, old information regarding the fight-or-flight theory has given way to updated research that demonstrates how men and women differ in their reactions during the stress response.

Emerging research indicates that while males tend to engage in more aggression-based responses to danger, females more often react with *tend and befriend* behaviors. These different reactions may be partly due to the differing effects of the hormone oxytocin on men and women. One study showed that oxytocin plays a key role in promoting a stronger sense of community and kinship for females, whereas for males, oxytocin may promote a clearer interpretation of competitive social interactions.[2] If a woman is under threat to herself or her child, the tend and befriend response enables her to instinctively gather her offspring and seek others nearby with whom she can band together to form a stronger defensive coalition.

In a traumatic HBC, a woman may look around her to see whom she can trust and who is on her side, or else she may desperately yearn to flee or defend herself and her baby from perceived threats to their survival. Regardless of the behavioral differences between the fight-or-flight and the tend and befriend responses, the well-documented physiological effects of the stress response have enormous implications for women undergoing stress and trauma throughout the labor and birth process.

The freeze response

When the fight-or-flight response fails to protect a person from acute danger, another adaptation called the *freeze response*, can serve as a last-ditch effort to preserve life. This response comes from the oldest, reptilian part of the brain and, like the fight-or-flight response, is instinctive. A person can enter the freeze response because she can't successfully flee, her attempts to fight the aggressor fail, or her brain instinctively registers that this danger is grave enough to bypass the fight-or-flight response altogether and move directly into the freeze response.

Before the freeze response takes hold, there is a moment when the intense energy generated by the body in the fight-or-flight response collides with the sudden onset of the freeze response and becomes trapped. According to Peter Levine, PhD, in *Waking the Tiger: Healing Trauma*, "The difference between the inner racing of the nervous system (engine), and the outer mobility (brake) of the body creates a forceful turbulence inside the

---

2   University of Haifa. (2013, July 31). 'Love hormone' oxytocin: Difference in social perception between men and women. *ScienceDaily*. Retrieved September 22, 2014 from www.sciencedaily.com/releases/2013/07/130731093257.htm.

body like a tornado.[3]" He likens this collision to the sensation of suddenly being interrupted while on the brink of sexual climax but magnified by 100 times. When this freeze occurs, the stored energy created from the freeze response must be fully discharged in order to complete the cycle of the stress response. If the energy is retained, it will remain in the person's body, potentially for many years, causing prolonged symptoms of trauma, such as recurrent flashbacks or nightmares.

For the woman in the intruder situation, the fight-or-flight response served her well by allowing her to jump out of bed and flee her home before harm could befall her. But imagine instead that she trips in the hallway and sees the intruder standing over her with a knife. As the woman's nervous system finds futility in escaping or defending against the attacker, the freeze response becomes dominant, and the following host of effects may occur in a matter of seconds:

- She becomes immobilized as her muscles lose all tone, and she lies limply on the floor.

- A feeling of serenity floods her as endorphins are released from her brain, and her pain threshold rises to greet the impending injury by the intruder, making her anticipated death less agonizing.

- Her blood pressure and heart rate drop and her breathing slows.

- Time stands still; numbness and confusion blanket her rational mind.

- No words come out when she opens her mouth to scream: she is mute.

- She may dissociate or undergo an altered state of consciousness where she feels detached, perhaps like she is looking down on her body from above.

- Her memory access and storage are impaired, and she will later have a difficult time recalling parts of the event.

---

3   Levine, P., Frederick, A. (1997). *Waking the Tiger: Healing Trauma.* Berkeley, CA: North Atlantic Books.

- The energy stored during the stress response becomes trapped in her body, her nerves retaining the adrenaline while simultaneously slowing her ability to react.

The freeze response is an altered state of consciousness, which evolved across all species of animals, including humans, for several different functions. First, the freeze response tricks the attacker into believing his victim is already dead, and in the case of animals, many predators will lose interest in already-dead prey since it poses a risk of being unfit to eat. Even a brief moment of inattention can grant the seemingly dead prey enough time to regain consciousness and flee the attack successfully. Second, the freeze response triggers the release of endorphins and causes mind-altering effects, which allow impending death to be less painful and terrifying. Some people who have experienced the freeze response say that they felt numb, calm, unaware of the passage of time, or they felt like they were floating outside their body. They can remain in this state of suspended animation until the nervous system detects that the danger has decreased or passed entirely.

When the woman in the intruder scenario finds safety—perhaps the intruder flees—she may find that she cannot control the shaking that wracks her body, and she begins to sob. This beneficial shaking, shivering, and sobbing allows her to discharge the energy trapped in her body during the stress response and to restore bodily processes to normal.

If she tries to suppress the shaking and sobbing as she calls 911, her body continues to store that energy, interlaced with the terrifying memories of the event, until discharge can occur. Levine writes, "the intense, frozen energy, instead of discharging, gets bound up with the overwhelming, highly activated, emotional states of terror, rage and helplessness.[4]" Levine suggests that humans, unlike other animals, cannot easily resolve their freeze response because of the terror involved in the event, which prolongs the trauma response and prevents resolution. That frozen energy can be stored for years causing suffering through recurrent memories, flashbacks, nightmares, and triggering events. However, discharge and resolution can occur when a person seeks therapy or other healing modalities to process the traumatic event.

---

4   Levine, P., Frederick, A. (1997). *Waking the Tiger: Healing Trauma*. Berkeley, CA: North Atlantic Books.

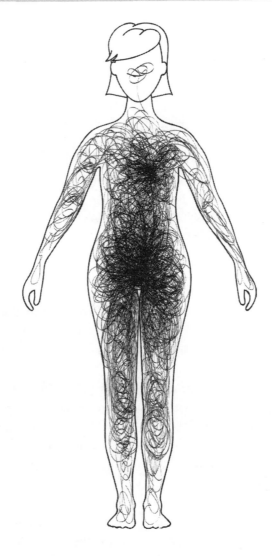

While appearing "normal" on the outside, a woman with stuck energy after the freeze response, if left untreated, may experience its aftereffects for a lifetime, with mental, emotional, and physical issues ranging from subtle to intense.

Kordenbrock, 2014

Polyvagal theory: How the brain reacts in trauma

To gain a better understanding of how a woman's mind and body cope with the extraordinary stress throughout an HBC, it can be helpful to examine how the human autonomic (or automatic, meaning not in our control) nervous system intertwines with our emotions and social behavior.

One way of explaining this complex system is with the polyvagal theory, developed by Stephen Porges, PhD Professor of Psychiatry, the Director of the Brain-Body Center at the University of Illinois, and the author of *The Polyvagal Theory: Neurophysiological Foundations of Emotions, Attachment, Communication, and Self-Regulation*. His theory hypothesizes that mammals are biologically and behaviorally driven by the need for safety and that the body has evolved hierarchical systems to ensure that survival mode is an automatic process, not mired in analysis and planning.[5]

Sarah Peyton, a neurobiologist educator, shares a concise explanation of how the polyvagal theory works within the framework of human emotion:

> There's a very large nerve bundle that runs in front of our spinal column called the vagus nerve. It's a regulator of how our body responds to the world in any given moment. When we feel safe and good, then we are in the forward-most channel of our nerves, and our body perceives that safety. This is when we are talkative, we laugh, and we have connection and empathy with others—it's when we are at our best.

> As soon as we receive messages of alarm, we begin to shift into fight-or-flight. When cortisol is released during fight-or-flight, our heart rates increase, we breathe more rapidly, and we lose our fine motor skills and ability to detect emotional nuance. Here we are driven to take action to try to survive.

> If our action to survive does not yield a good result, we move into the freeze response, situated in the dorsal or rearmost channel of the vagus bundle. There is a decrease in heart rate, blood pressure, and respiration, and the traveling speed of nervous system messages decreases one-hundredfold. We are simply trying to conserve life when we move into this state. When this happens, it is almost impossible to integrate emotions, because our nervous system is not responding quickly enough

---

5   Dykema, R, (Interviewer) & Porges, S. (Interviewee). (2006). *How your nervous system sabotages your ability to relate: An interview with Stephen Porges about his polyvagal theory*. Retrieved September 22, 2014 from http://www.nexuspub.com/articles_2006/interview_porges_06_ma.phphttp://www.nexuspub.com/articles_2006/interview_porges_06_ma.php

to be able to name or resonate with the various experiences that are happening to us. Freeze is the home of shock, dissociation, confusion, and shame.

While the fight-or-flight and freeze responses guide the biological actions of humans in life-threatening situations, the polyvagal theory clarifies how those responses affect a person's emotions and ability to connect with others during and after the event. This helps to explain why HBC women have difficulty remembering the chronological details of their births or why they perceived that their birth team seemed so angry with them.

The fallout from life-threatening events

While the fight-or-flight and freeze responses are life-preserving efforts in an acutely dangerous situation, the effects of the stress response and the physiologic repercussions can last well beyond the point at which the body resumes its state of homeostasis (return to normal functioning). For example, after the intruder incident, the woman may continue to be deeply shaken. She may avoid returning to her home, feeling her safety has been jeopardized. Intrusive thoughts or images of the incident may infiltrate her mind while she is trying to focus on other tasks. When she sits at her computer and her mind replays the scene in her head, she may notice that her heart rate quickens and once again a cold sweat trickles from her armpits, just as she experienced on that terrifying night. Although she is now safe, she feels traumatized by the event and is powerless to regain her sense of wholeness or to capture a feeling of security that she had before the incident.

"Trauma is any experience that the brain has a hard time integrating," says Peyton. "It includes unresolved feelings, distress, and mourning about an unexpected experience. The person who experiences the event determines whether or not it was traumatic, which is based on how the experience lives in that person afterwards."

How the stress response affects labor and birth

In an uncomplicated birth, a woman is exquisitely adapted to integrate the changes in her body that each new stage of labor brings. As she moves through labor, her hormones mobilize to free stored glucose and take in extra oxygen to allow her uterus to contract while supporting her baby.

Powerful endorphins are released by the pituitary and hypothalamus glands, helping the woman cope with the intensity of each contraction. The mother and baby work together as the baby moves lower into the pelvis, and the mother's pushing effort supplements the uterus's robust contractions. When the baby emerges, he is ready to transition to life outside the womb, and hormones prompt him to begin breathing spontaneously as his mother reaches down to grasp his body. The new mother's attention is shifted to her newborn, and the two begin the dance of nursing. The woman's body then receives a hormonal signal that the placenta is ready to be born, and contractions help release the placenta from her uterus, which now constricts to control bleeding.

The delicate balance of the labor hormones, including oxytocin, along with the mother's emotional wellbeing and a strong need for privacy and safety, combine to form a healthy birthing environment that does not activate the stress response. When this delicate balance is upset, the mother may nose-dive straight into the fight-or-flight or freeze response. This stress response can cause labor to become unproductive and can result in great suffering and distress for the woman and her baby, during birth, in the postpartum time, and possibly for years to come.

Of course women planning to give birth in the hospital are not immune to conditions that prompt the stress responses. Even a woman who is quite comfortable with medical staff, interventions, and a lack of privacy can find herself suddenly plunged into the stress response by a threat to her or her baby's health, or by an unexpected cesarean. However, the woman planning a hospital birth typically has some degree of ease with being in the hospital, or, at the very least, she is aware that she will encounter numerous interventions and strangers. The mother planning a hospital birth is prepared to be in the hospital and is more likely to have toured the labor and delivery unit, taken a hospital-based childbirth preparation class, or hired a doula for extra support. In addition, she will not perceive the shift from being at home to arriving at the hospital as such a fear-invoking experience since it was her plan from the beginning.

The fight-or-flight or freeze response, so precisely evolved to ensure survival of the species, can upset the balance needed to maintain a healthy labor pattern and can cause contractions to cease or malfunction. When a laboring mother becomes fearful or anxious, the oxytocin feedback loop that caused her strong and efficient contractions short-circuits, and contractions become colicky and non-progressive. The endorphins that bolstered her ability to cope with her intense contractions are replaced by catecholamines, which interrupt the flow of oxytocin, slowing her labor and making her contractions weak and ineffectual. Lactic acid build-up in her large uterine muscle causes increasing pain and fatigue. The baby, previously content within his mother's squeezing uterus, now begins to feel the effects of the stress hormones flooding the placenta and restricting blood flow, and he reacts with a slowing of his heart. The laboring woman's nervous system receives the clear signal that giving birth under these circumstances is unsafe, and her progress may stop entirely. The laboring woman is now terrified of what might happen to her and her unborn child. The people surrounding the mother grow more alarmed as time passes, noting that the baby is in distress and the mother's vital signs are now concerning as well, with steadily climbing blood pressure and heart rate. Their worried looks and hushed whispers convey that something is drastically wrong.

Risk factors for birth trauma

Although any woman has the potential to suffer psychological trauma during her birth, some pre-existing risk factors make trauma more likely to occur. It is important to understand that risk factors do not cause birth trauma but are merely indicators that should be taken into careful consideration when assessing a woman's likelihood for experiencing birth trauma.

All pregnant women and partners need preparation for a potential cesarean, but for women with pre-existing risk factors, the chances of emotional trauma resulting from an unwanted cesarean are even higher. When the birth team has ample time to discuss risk factors and how these factors apply to a homebirth cesarean, women and their birth teams can develop a comprehensive plan for professional mental health support and cultivate a strong awareness of her needs during labor and birth.

> In my opinion, one of the biggest risk factors for a traumatic HBC is refusal to learn about cesarean prenatally and to accept it as potential birth outcome. I remember reluctantly doing the hospital tour and walking past the OR dismissively, refusing to acknowledge it even existed. The truth was, I was so terrified

of ending up in there that it made me nauseous. But instead of dealing with that fear and releasing it, I stuffed it down. It resurfaced during my HBC in all its ugliness.
—Laurie (2008/HBC, 2010/HBAC; Southern U.S.)

While no formula exists to fully predict which women will suffer trauma related to a homebirth cesarean, we asked HBC mothers, birth workers, and mental health professionals for their help in compiling a list of risk factors, in no particular order, which may predispose women to HBC trauma. Some risk factors have been well researched for birth trauma, such as clinical depression in pregnancy, while others have been revealed by HBC mothers and birth professionals as significant contributors to their own, or their clients' HBC trauma. Women and their care providers should understand that risk factors for a traumatic HBC range widely and may apply to most pregnant and birthing women:

- Women with a strong need for maintaining control

- Magical thinkers (women unwilling to consider less-than-optimal outcomes)

- Lack of preparation for various birth outcomes, or dismissal of the possibility of cesarean

- Women who describe themselves as Type A

- Rigid or unrealistic expectations for birth/self/birth team

- People-pleasers/women who struggle with setting clear boundaries

- Viewing the hospital system or medical staff as villains

- Fear of hospitals, doctors, medical workers

- Depression, anxiety, or other mental health disorders

- Experience of traumatic events during pregnancy

- History of unresolved trauma of any type, including neglect, witnessing violence, abandonment, and/or negative medical experiences

- Unhealthy/abusive relationships, past or present

- Sexual abuse survivors

- Poor social support structure

While some of these risk factors have a clear relationship to birth trauma, others are more difficult to comprehend, such as the tendency to be people pleasers. Imagine a woman who strives to please others and is often unable to assert her own needs. She didn't reveal a history of trauma or abuse to her birth team in her prenatal care but did note that her relationship with her mother is troubled. Undergoing a homebirth cesarean, this woman may tell her birth team that she is coping well with the change in plans, and they perceive that they are meeting her needs. Internally, she is struggling and desperately wants her partner, her midwife, or her doula to advocate on her behalf, but that does not happen. In her mind, she is back in the exam room where, as a teenager, she was abusively treated by the doctor conducting her first well-woman exam, as her mother stood nearby, mutely watching. This flashback unfolds as the woman lies immobile, the doctor repeatedly performing rough vaginal exams without permission, her partner standing passively by the bed. The woman's history of unprocessed medical abuse, layered with other risk factors, such as a lack of support and her inability to assert her own needs, places her at higher risk of experiencing her HBC as traumatic.

According to Penny Simkin, author of *When Survivors Give Birth: Understanding and Healing the Effects of Early Sexual Abuse on Childbearing Women,* women have many reasons for not sharing information about past abuse: "they may have no memory of it; they may believe it would be futile and embarrassing; they may believe it has no relevance; they may believe they have healed and it no longer affects them.[6]" In such cases, the midwife or doula can reiterate why she thinks

---

6   Simkin, P., & Klaus, P. (2004). *When Survivors Give Birth: Understanding and Healing the Effects of Early Sexual Abuse on Childbearing Women.* Seattle, WA: Classic Day Publishing.

disclosure will ultimately be helpful for the woman and then offer her referrals for counseling or therapy.

Some pregnant women may not understand that there can be a link between their history or personality and potential birth trauma. A woman may wonder why her midwife asks her to provide information she has not shared with other healthcare providers, and why it might help to reveal her history. If the woman has a clear understanding of why the midwife is inquiring about her past and current experiences and that she is linking it to her risk for birth trauma, she may be more invested in the ensuing conversations.

History of abuse as a risk factor for HBC trauma
Women are often survivors of physical, emotional, and psychological abuse in childhood and/or adulthood. Many women were abused by a parent or other adult in childhood, or they have been the victim of rape or assault by a partner, acquaintance, or stranger. According to the World Health Organization, "recent global prevalence figures indicate that 35% of women worldwide have experienced either intimate partner violence or non-partner sexual violence in their lifetime.[7]" Women can also be victimized in non-sexual ways, such as in a violent robbery, by witnessing violence, or by experiencing abuse at the hands of a medical professional who performs procedures against her will.

For some of these women, out-of-hospital birth offers the option of maintaining control over their bodies during the overwhelming process of birth. Women might choose to work with midwives in order to retain autonomy over their choices and feel that a midwife will compassionately meet their needs throughout the childbearing year. Women who have been victims of sexual assault and/or violence may have a difficult time trusting others, and feel that a midwife is their safest option to walk through birth with them.

---

7   World Health Organization. (2013). Global and regional estimates of violence against women: prevalence and health effects of intimate partner violence and non-partner sexual violence. Geneva, Switzerland: World Health Organization. Retrieved from http://apps.who.int/iris/bitstream/10665/85239/1/9789241564625_eng.pdf?ua=1

I'm a sexual assault survivor. As my son's birth sits in my memory, I see now how much of my HBC trauma was tied to issues about that part of my life.
—JODY (2011/HBC, WESTERN U.S.)

I worked hard with a therapist, doula, and my midwife to address everything I could think of concerning my abuse history. We talked about different scenarios, what to do if I started having flashbacks or anxiety and how they should take care of me if we ended up in a transport.
—EMMA (2013/HBC, WESTERN U.S.)

In their book *Traumatic Childbirth*, Beck, Driscoll, and Watson report that for women who have been victims of sexual abuse, particularly in childhood, labor and birth present several opportunities for them to be re-traumatized. First, they note that "typical interventions or events that occur during labor and delivery may act as triggers to their abuse.[8]" Vaginal exams, the presence of authority figures when feeling exposed and vulnerable, and even the sensation of the baby moving through the birth canal can trigger powerful traumatic memories for women in labor.

Next, Beck, Driscoll, and Watson describe that messages conveyed by healthcare providers that encourage women to comply with instructions throughout birth can inadvertently cause harm to a woman who may have heard similar phrases from her abuser. A woman who was raped as a child may have been told to lie down and hold still. Hearing these words in the midst of an already out-of-control HBC can cause her to spiral deeper into the stress response, resulting in trauma.

Finally, the authors observe that "having some control in labor is not only important for women but is paramount for women who are survivors of childhood sexual abuse. Often, women who have suffered abuse may equate powerlessness, helplessness, and loss of control with being abused.[9]" In a homebirth cesarean, the unforeseen shift from a trusted birth team to a crew of hospital staff who are strangers, can mean greater potential for a traumatic birth.

---

8   Beck, C.T., Driscoll, J.W., & Watson, S . (2013) *Traumatic Childbirth*. New York, NY: Routledge.

9   Beck, C.T., Driscoll, J.W., & Watson, S . (2013) *Traumatic Childbirth*. New York, NY: Routledge.

Prenatal assessment for birth trauma risk factors

At the onset of care with a new client, the midwife and doula can begin assessing for risk factors in a variety of ways. All women need to be screened early in prenatal care for a history of trauma, as well as for pre-pregnancy and current perinatal mood and anxiety disorders (PMADs) such as depression or anxiety. The woman's medical history will contain information about her health challenges, and it must include questions about mental health disorders, substance abuse, prior medical procedures, abuse, and trauma.

The woman's partner, or accompanying friend or family member, may occasionally disclose information that the woman herself has forgotten or does not want to share with her birth team. When this disclosure occurs, the midwife or doula can shift her focus back to the mother, and ask her if she wants to explain or address anything about what has just been revealed, allowing the client to regain control of the discussion as she feels comfortable.

One way to begin the discussion about prior trauma is to request that a client fill out a questionnaire. Elizabeth Davis designed the Mother's Confidential Worksheet, available in her book, *Heart & Hands, A Midwife's Guide to Pregnancy and Birth, 5th edition*, which asks about the woman's history of rape, abuse, and trauma.[10] Davis explains, "It's a way to begin conversation around trauma, and to look at mechanisms for getting deep down to where those traumas are lodged in order to find ways to release them before the birth." Unlike a general health history that becomes part of the mother's permanent record, the midwife makes clear that she will read and return the confidential worksheet to the mother and it will not go into her chart.

Midwives are sometimes uncomfortable addressing a personal history of abuse or trauma with a family member or partner present. The woman may not have told her partner about her history, she might be experiencing abuse in her current relationship, or she might feel unsafe or reluctant about sharing it in her prenatal appointments in front of another person. Some women will simply need time and preparation to broach the subject with a partner or their birth team.

---

10   Davis, E. (2012). *Heart & Hands, A Midwife's Guide to Pregnancy and Birth, 5th edition.* New York, NY. Ten Speed Press.

Elizabeth Davis suggests that the midwife can protect a woman's emotional safety and privacy by telling her clients at the initial visit that she always schedules the 16- or 20-week appointment as one where the mother comes alone. (See Appendix D, Schedule of Mental Health, Transport, and Cesarean Topics.) During this solo visit, the midwife can frankly address the mother's confidential worksheet and make a plan to revisit any issues throughout pregnancy and in the postpartum period. The midwife can also ask the woman about her comfort level in addressing her history in front of her partner and others who might accompany her to appointments.

For some women, openly discussing their history of trauma with their birth team will be enough for them to move forward with a deeper sense of connection and trust in their upcoming birth experience. For many other women, however, it will be helpful to seek the care of a mental health professional who can listen without judgment, and who will provide constructive coping mechanisms to integrate prior traumatic experiences that may affect labor and birth, particularly if a cesarean is needed. The midwife or doula can make referrals for mental health professionals who specialize in caring for women through pregnancy, birth, and afterwards. Once referrals have been made, it is important for the birth professional to follow up with the client and discuss how the treatment is going for the woman, and if further or different referrals are needed.

When a midwife sorts through her client's health history and learns more about the mother's potential risk factors, she can begin to dialogue about how these aspects of the woman's mental, physical, and emotional health might affect her pregnancy, the birth experience, and her transition to parenting a new baby. For example, a woman might describe that while she was not physically abused as a child, she did witness the abuse of her mother and siblings and she thinks that has made it difficult for her to assert her needs throughout her life. She might also mention that she has never spent time in a hospital but has mistrust for the medical system in general and wants to avoid going to the hospital at all costs. Her midwife might observe that when she describes a typical transport scenario to the woman in a prenatal visit, the mother shifts uncomfortably in her seat and is unable to make eye contact.

The midwife may reflect what she notices in the woman's body language and ask how they can address the topic of hospital transports and cesareans in a way that would be respectful to the woman's individual needs. The midwife can also clearly explain the relevance of discussing risk factors for traumatic birth and HBC trauma.

The job of the midwife and doula, who are not therapists, is to safely open the door to honest discussion in a variety of ways, verbal and written. They can then normalize trauma risk factors and mention that many women have complex combinations of events and challenges in the past that put them at risk for birth trauma, and reassure their clients that they can safely discuss their feelings and history with the birth team. Midwives and doulas can also tell mothers that they screen all clients, which can prevent mothers from feeling singled out. However, if a woman chooses not to divulge important information, the birth team may never discover it and the client holds the responsibility for that.

When a pregnant woman who has previously experienced trauma receives thoughtful care from her birth team and an experienced mental health professional, she can feel a sense of wholeness and resolution, which can greatly benefit her as she begins motherhood. The birth team can also begin to understand the individual needs, hopes, and expectations of the woman, and in return they can clarify their own roles in supporting her emotional needs during her labor, birth, and postpartum.

HBC trauma: Julie's birth

Julie had a planned hospital birth with her first child, and although the birth itself was medically uncomplicated, she experienced her doctor dismissing her requests, doing vaginal exams without permission, and pushing her to accept an epidural. She described her birth experience as one of feeling powerless and bullied. During her next pregnancy, she planned a homebirth, hoping to avoid a repeat of her first birth situation, and she built a relationship with a midwife who reassured her that she would be treated respectfully by her birth team.

During her labor, Julie was caught off-guard by how quickly her contractions intensified. She could feel herself becoming triggered by the trauma from her previous birth, causing her to shriek with the intensity of her contractions. Her midwife arrived shortly after labor began, and she proceeded to check Julie's vital signs and the baby's heart rate. Concerned the baby might be breech, the midwife hurriedly donned gloves, asking to perform a vaginal exam without explaining her suspicions. Julie simply nodded consent as the next contraction began. As the midwife checked her cervix, Julie's body shifted into panic mode. Her breathing became shallow, her heart pounded, and she began to shake uncontrollably. Distracted by the task at hand, the midwife was unaware of Julie's shift into the stress response.

Finding a foot protruding into Julie's vagina, the midwife immediately moved into emergency mode, called 911, and contacted the OB/GYN on staff to prepare for a cesarean upon Julie's arrival. The apprentice, inexperienced in transport situations, left Julie alone to pack clothing and other items for her. Ryan, Julie's husband, seemed paralyzed with shock and was unable to connect with Julie or support her as the paramedics arrived. As stress hormones flooded her body, Julie was alone in struggling with the deep work of her painful contractions, fighting the urge to push, and attempting to comprehend what was happening. There was no opportunity to wrap her mind around this sudden change of plans.

At the hospital, the medical team descended on Julie, and her midwife was pushed aside to make room for emergency cesarean preparations. Ryan, still dazed by what was happening, stood silently aside. The obstetrician thrust his fingers into Julie's vagina, neither preparing her nor seeking consent. As this happened, Julie's heart raced and her breathing quickened. She felt like a caged animal and longed to escape the nightmare that was unfolding. Looking around the room for support, she finally made eye contact with her midwife, but nurses quickly rolled Julie onto her side, facing her away from her midwife, who was trying to reach for her hand. A cold needle punctured her back as the anesthesiologist administered the anesthetic medication needed for surgery.

As she was wheeled to the operating room, Julie's mind numbed and she became disoriented. Her body felt like it was separated from her psyche, floating above the gurney. Although surrounded by six masked nurses and doctors, Julie had a sense that she was completely alone, and nobody else existed in that moment. The rest of the cesarean was a blur, pierced only by the crying of her baby.

Surgery as trauma

Women's health physical therapist Tami Lynn Kent suggests that all cesareans are traumatic to the body, whether on the emotional, physical, spiritual, or cellular levels. "It doesn't matter if the cesarean is elective or an HBC; the body experiences surgery as a traumatic event even though it may be necessary," says Kent. "In some ways, we are still wild creatures and surgery causes a physical separation of muscle and tissue, which the body responds to as traumatic."

Delving deeper into the concept of surgery as trauma, Levine, in his book *Waking the Tiger: Healing Trauma*, explains the concept of surgery as trauma:

> Even though a person may recognize that an operation is necessary... as the surgeon cuts through flesh, muscle, and bone, it still registers in the body as a life-threatening event. On the "cellular level" the body perceives that it has sustained a wound serious enough to place it in mortal danger. When trauma is concerned, the perception of the instinctual nervous system carries more weight—much more. This biological fact is a primary reason why surgery will often produce a post-traumatic reaction.[11]

Ann, whose story we share throughout this book, says that even though she was awake for her cesarean, her body and mind were in different places. "My rational mind was aware that the surgery wasn't life-threatening," she says. "While my higher mind held those thoughts, my body perceived that it was being physically constrained like a zebra under a hungry lion. I was torn open, in what, under any other circumstances, would be a killing blow."

While the nervous system perceives all surgery as a threat to survival and while HBC mothers experience the emotional loss of their intended birth, these mothers may experience an amplified sense that they are dying or close to death. Midwife Sister MorningStar notes that: "Cesarean is different from other surgeries because it is unique to the maternal woman. The sacred life force that carries our drive to protect, preserve, and nurture our

---

11   Levine, P., Frederick, A. (1997). *Waking the Tiger: Healing Trauma.* Berkeley, CA: North Atlantic Books

babies is at a heightened level during labor and birth. That awareness is not put to sleep during surgery."

Many women report feeling disintegration in their mind, body, and spirit during their surgical birth experience. Even though Ann thought she was dying during her cesarean, she told herself not to cry for fear of being labeled hysterical. "I remember lying there thinking that I had survived a violent mother, a rape, depression, and eating disorders, but this was the thing that was going to break me," she says. "I had a vision of my soul curling into a tiny mammalian ball, getting smaller and smaller and drying up like a grape turning into a raisin. I knew I would never come back from this. It felt like everyone else was in the living world and I was passing into a shadow place. They would take my baby and go on, and I would be left alone to pass away."

HBC trauma

In a homebirth cesarean, things can happen really fast. Women are in the care of medical staff, and they often feel abandoned by their birth team. Most women in the hospital feel a loss of control, and like everything is being done to them, not in collaboration with them. In this time of crisis, women are flooded with fear and that can trigger old memories of fear and being out of control.
—KAREN JACKSON FORBES, PSYCHOTHERAPIST, WESTERN U.S.

While the stress response is an instinctual reaction to perceived danger, trauma is the severe emotional distress that results after the incident. Women who planned to give birth at home or in a birth center, but who are transported to the hospital for a cesarean, often report experiencing both the stress response during the birth and emotional trauma afterwards.

Wendy Davis, PhD, psychotherapist and executive director of Postpartum Support International, describes birth trauma as:

the experience of having something happen that is so disturbing and disruptive to a person's psyche that they feel that their sense of wholeness is threatened. That can be psychological, physical, or spiritual. Birth trauma can be experienced by the woman birthing the baby, the partner, and the care provider. But specifically, it isn't just that the birth is experienced as painful and stressful. There is almost always some pain and distress with giving birth, but the trauma is about shattered expectations about birth, or the sense of safety as deeply disrupted.

The following list outlines the four most common elements we discovered from interviewing women who describe their HBCs as traumatic.

1) Grief over the loss of a dream

According to neurobiology educator Sarah Peyton, one of the causes of trauma in a homebirth cesarean is that women first grieve the loss of their long-anticipated homebirth dream, and then that dream gives way to a cold, impersonal surgical birth experience. This results in an insurmountable sense of trauma for some women in the weeks and possibly years following their HBC. For a woman who spent months envisioning an intimate birth in the privacy of her home or familiarity of a birth center, the transition to the hospital, and then the operating room, represents a harsh dismissal of everything she had longed for in her birth experience.

My HBC represented the death of a dream. This was going to be our last baby and we wanted as many of our children present and participating as possible. I wanted them to see how beautiful natural childbirth is. And we got the opposite. They saw me traumatized.
—JULIA (2002, 2004, 2008/HOSPITAL BIRTH, 2006, 2011/HB, 2013/HBC; CANADA)

2) Sense of powerlessness and helplessness

Another component of trauma in an HBC, Peyton explains, is that "women mourn when they are not in power, when they are helpless and not allowed to have choices about what is happening to them." The layering of the profound loss of a dream with the loss of one's own choice can cause great suffering. One of the strengths of homebirth is that women and their partners are presented with choices in their care, valuing the opportunity to discuss and clarify options, and then they make choices without the heavy hand of an authority figure pressing on them. When homebirth women become merely another medical patient in the hospital, they may feel helpless or unskilled in negotiating for their choices or feel that they are not treated as capable decision-makers.

When this experience of powerlessness is compounded by physical restrictions and immobilization, the sense of helplessness grows exponentially. Scot Nichols, a somatic psychotherapist, explains that "with cesarean birth there is anesthetization, so you can't fight and you can't flee. You can't even think your way through it. The cognitive functions are shutting down and the body is going into red alert." This is the body's final effort to conserve life after the fight-or-flight response fails. During a cesarean, it results in women being unable to assert their needs, even on a basic level, since communication is nearly impossible in the freeze response.

When I was in the hospital after the cesarean, I was so exhausted, trauma-tized, and half-crazy with new mama hormones, I had a deep sense of being a trapped, vulnerable animal.
—ANN (2011/HBC, MIDWESTERN U.S.)

3) Fear for the safety of self and/or baby's survival

The loss of a dream and a sense of powerlessness are major components in creating the perfect storm leading to birth trauma. These pieces can be further exacerbated by a heightened sense of alarm, or the laboring woman's fear for her own safety and/or her baby's survival. Although a mother's life may not actually be threatened, if she perceives it as such or if she is worried that her baby might die, her brain interprets the danger signals as real and immediate threats, prompting her body to move into survival mode and her mind to interpret the event as life-threatening.

The surgeon nicked my bladder and said I lost a lot of blood. It was in that moment that I panicked—I thought this was where I was going to die. I kept saying I was going to die.
—KORIN (2006, 2012/HBC; WESTERN U.S.)

I wasn't able to swallow and breathe on the table. I thought I was dying.
—ERIN (2009/HBC, 2012/HBAC; WESTERN U.S.)

My words weren't forming right, I couldn't speak. I had no idea that trembling was normal and not life-threatening. I thought I was going to die.
—DANA (2012/HBC, WESTERN U.S.)

They said her heart rate had not recovered, so we were going to the theatre
(operating room). I was put to sleep for her birth, and I went under thinking
she would be dead.
—JADE (2012/HBC, UNITED KINGDOM)

4) Profound sense of aloneness or abandonment

According to Wendy Davis, "Trauma is usually experienced when someone feels deeply alone, and there exists the terror of 'no one can help me' even if someone is holding you, you feel psychologically and spiritually bereft. That's why some people experience trauma even if their partner or midwife is right there." For many women we interviewed, their experience of isolation, regardless of the support surrounding them, was a critical component of their deep trauma.

A laboring woman may feel increasingly vulnerable and dependent on others to provide physical, mental, and spiritual support as her labor progresses. She may begin to seek reassurance from her birth team that her pain is a normal sign of progress. When the pregnancy or labor becomes unexpectedly complicated and she is transported to the hospital, she needs the unflinching presence of her birth team and support people. When the people she relies on most are missing, distracted, unaware, or unsure how to provide for her needs, she feels desperately alone, even in their presence.

I felt abandoned and was treated as though I was less than human. Instead of
holding my hand during the birth, my midwife talked with the surgeon about
their weekend.
—CHRISTINE (2009, 2012/HBC; NORTHEASTERN U.S.)

The fallout from the freeze response during an HBC

During a homebirth cesarean, when a woman transitions into the freeze stress response, several adaptations take place that can cause her to have a lasting sense of trauma. Some commonly reported repercussions of the freeze response are an inability to understand and connect with others in the moment, memory loss, replaying of traumatic events, and a deep sense of shame.

When a woman moves into the stress response, her limbic system, or the social interaction center of her brain, loses its ability to accurately discern the emotions and facial expressions of those around her. So much interpersonal communication is based on humans' ability to not only hear the speaker's words but also to interpret their body language and facial expressions to add meaning and context. At a time where she has lost her ability to understand subtle body language and emotional nuance, she will perceive that her partner, the hospital staff, and the birth team are angry, unsupportive, or even a threat to her survival. Her nervous system is driving her survival mode, constantly evaluating the safety level of the people surrounding her. This primitive instinct allows her nervous system to avoid danger, yet it interferes with her need to feel connected to, and trusting of, those around her. Her brain shuts down or freezes in response, and this mechanism, meant to save her life, reaffirms her worst fear—that nobody is there to help her after all. Later, she might struggle to understand why the people surrounding her seemed to be judging her or appeared angry, because that is what she will recall.

Porges writes in his book on the polyvagal theory that in this state of perceived danger, "neutral faces appear to be angry, so you misread everything as it relates to survival. Your nervous system evaluates anything that may be neutral as dangerous, rather than pleasant.[12]"

Another by-product of the freeze response is the way traumatic events are encoded as memories in the brain. The storage of memories can be categorized as either explicit or implicit. Explicit memories, stored in the brain's hippocampus, are pieces of information that people consciously recall—locations of certain items, phone numbers, calendar dates, and events. Implicit memories, written in the amygdala, are subconscious, procedural recollections of tasks such as driving a car, tying a shoe, sensory recollections, or how a beloved grandmother's house smelled during childhood. Implicit memories are closely tied to emotions, which can explain why a person may automatically feel happy and secure when encountering the smell from their grandmother's home.

---

12 Dykema, R, (Interviewer) & Porges, S. (Interviewee). (2006). *How your nervous system sabotages your ability to relate: An interview with Stephen Porges about his polyvagal theory.* Retrieved September 22, 2014 from http://www.nexuspub.com/articles_2006/interview_porges_06_ma.phphttp://www.nexuspub.com/articles_2006/interview_porges_06_ma.php

During a traumatic HBC, the memory-storage process is interrupted. Peyton explains: "The part of the brain that stores explicit memory shuts down. It's like the fuse gets blown for the hippocampus, and the part of the brain that writes down clear autobiographical memory goes offline. However, the amygdala remains online and continues to record emotional memory, even if these women don't remember what happened.

> *Days later I didn't remember my midwife visiting me in the hospital. My husband told me she was there, but I had no memory of her visit.*
> —BETH (2009/HBC, WESTERN U.S.)

> *I lost many memories from the time I first heard the word "breech" because I was in complete shock. Some of it was my body's way of protecting me.*
> —JULIA (2002, 2004, 2008/HOSPITAL BIRTH, 2006, 2011/HB, 2013/HBC; CANADA)

For some women, one moment during the cesarean becomes engrained in their memory and automatically gets replayed over and over again. "People can get stuck in time, re-experiencing trauma. This is just how memory works." Peyton continues, "The hippocampus, the part of the brain that integrates, tracks, and timestamps memory, needs to have the trauma resolved. The way that the brain can be helped to resolve this trauma is by calming the woman's body in the presence of whatever memory remains explicitly available, and instilling feelings of safety, so that the hippocampus can be released to focus on recreating, reconstructing, and understanding the timestamps."

When memories of an HBC are deeply distressing and traumatic, a mother can have great difficulty moving forward to seek resolution and peace with her experience. For some women who experience a traumatic HBC, healing will come in working with a mental health professional, bodyworker, or other care provider who can offer tools for coping with the physical sensations that the memories evoke, guiding the mother through discharging energy stored from the freeze stress response.

Another element of the fallout from the freeze response is the sense of shame that women commonly report. Women say that they felt ashamed that they could not birth their babies vaginally, ashamed at how they behaved in a certain moment in labor, or felt shamed by a hospital staff member or their midwife for something they did or said.

After I consented to the cesarean, I felt like I had absolutely failed. I had so much shame that I couldn't give birth vaginally. I couldn't do it how my mom had done it. I couldn't give my daughter the birth that I wanted her to have.
—DANA (2012/HBC, WESTERN U.S.)

In a sense, "shame serves an important function in the evolution of mammals as social creatures," says Nichols. "If your child runs across the street and you can't grab him with your hand, you can verbally shame him through a harsh 'Noooo!' That shame will freeze the nervous system because belonging to a group for a young mammal is imperative for survival. If that belonging gets threatened, the child is going to freeze in their tracks and find out what is going on. Shame contracts our energy system."

A laboring woman in the process of a homebirth cesarean is vulnerable to the reactions and words of others, and her own sense of shame may peak just when she needs affirmation and reassurance the most. A woman having a pre-labor HBC due to complications in pregnancy can also have this same sense of shame. HBC mother Jaime says, "I never went into labor, and to me, that feels even more shameful. My body couldn't even get to that preliminary stage of giving birth."

Calming the alarm response during an HBC

Women react to the distress of a homebirth cesarean in varying ways and degrees. Our initial hard-wired impulse, as in the tend-and-befriend response, is to want to connect with those around us, regardless of the situation. Experts we interviewed, including Scot Nichols, Wendy Davis, and Sarah Peyton, outlined four ideas that birth team members, partners, and hospital staff can use to support the woman throughout her birth experience. We have organized these suggestions into the four points of centering—connect, touch, ask, narrate—for calming the mother's alarm response. Birth professionals can use these tools when women are in need of extra support. Childbirth educators can also teach these life skills to partners so they can practice supporting the mother beyond the birth.

1. **Connect**
   Connection begins with vocal pacing and body language awareness when speaking to a mother. The support person must speak slowly and clearly, in a low pitch, with calm tones whenever a mother appears to be

experiencing the stress response. When the woman is frantic or terrified, the support person can use simple terms and descriptions. As the woman calms, the support person can follow the woman's lead, resuming a more normal conversational tone. Using this vocal pacing is helpful with calming the stress response by sending her brain the message that, in the midst of chaos, she is supported. Maintaining eye contact and giving gentle looks of appreciation and warmth also convey reassurance and openness. If the birth team senses that eye contact is too intense for the mother, they can avert their eyes periodically while still providing support. The midwife or doula who is more bonded with the mother can provide this support, sitting by her side rather than standing above her in a way that the mother might interpret as threatening.

2. **Touch**

The offer of physical touch to the laboring woman is vital. With the mother's permission, the partner, doula, or midwife can gently stroke the mother's leg, arm, or back, which helps her remain connected and attuned to her supporters. If the mother is experiencing the stress response, this touch allows her autonomic nervous system to identify the person touching her as an ally. Sometimes, as a result of feeling overwhelmed at the least, or traumatized at the worst, the mother may need her support person to verbalize that she is touching her so that she can better perceive that touch: "I'm right here. My hand is on your leg." Reassuring touch can help the mother feel safe and enable her to better hear what her support person is saying.

3. **Ask**

Throughout the transport and hospital experience the support team can ask the mother simple questions: "How are you breathing? What kind of emotions are you feeling?" If she expresses fear, the support person can ask her what she is afraid of and validate her feelings with warmth and comfort rather than blindly reassuring her that she is safe. Reassurance of attentiveness, presence, and continued care is also important.

4. Narrate

As events in a homebirth cesarean unfold, women may feel confused in the fog of intense emotions, labor hormones, the stress response, fatigue, and medications. It's helpful for mothers feeling overwhelmed or in trauma to have the situation explained to them in simple terms. Davis says, "If her birth team gives her clear information about what is happening in the room, with her baby and her body, her brain has a chance to come back into balance and turn the fight-or-flight emergency system off."

We all need to know details about our environment in order to feel safe. For a woman who has prior trauma or is in trauma during labor, it's helpful for her to have one person who can stay close and ask open-ended questions like "Would you like me to tell you what's going on?" Then tell her, "We are in the hospital, considering the possibility of a cesarean. Your baby's heart rate is slow but still recovering well."

"If you've never gone through trauma yourself," says Wendy Davis, "or you've never helped someone else through trauma, this kind of support may not come naturally. It's something that a lot of people need to practice in order to have the skills at the ready when trauma is taking place."

In addition to using the four points of centering, the midwife or doula can also stay connected by describing what she is experiencing in her own body, says Sarah Peyton. "The midwife might say 'I am feeling so much warmth for you. You can hear my voice and you can hear me asking about you and your baby.'" Peyton continues "This narration lets the mother know that emotional support still exists in the middle of all of the technological interventions, and it will give the mother a sense of being connected."

It's important that the birth team never blindly reassure a woman by telling her that she is safe. She may perceive her experience as the worst thing that could ever happen and therefore the furthest thing from safe. Trying to calm her by telling her she is safe may spiral her into deeper trauma through the belief that her support people are unaware of or ignoring her true feelings. Instead, narrating the actual events of the situation will help ground her in the experience.

With practice, such as by role-playing with other birth professionals and hands-on experience, midwives and doulas can learn how to stay connected with a mother during an HBC and be comfortable offering physical touch in times of stress, know when to ask questions, and how to narrate the situation. These skills may help alleviate a crisis or prevent the mother from plunging into the stress response, resulting in profound birth trauma.

PTSD: The long-term fallout from traumatic HBC

When a mother has a homebirth cesarean, the psychological and emotional effects last well beyond the time she leaves the hospital. If the birth was traumatic for her, she may suffer post-traumatic stress disorder (PTSD), sometimes in addition to perinatal mood and anxiety disorders (PMADs). To understand how these different disorders affect HBC women, it is important to clarify what they are and how they are distinct from each other. (See Chapter 10 for more information on PMADs, PTSD, and screening tools for birth professionals.) When women understand that their birth trauma can exist alongside other mental health challenges, such as postpartum anxiety, they can seek help from a mental health professional experienced in both postpartum PTSD and PMADs.

Some women will experience a combination of these disorders following birth, and others will suffer symptoms specific to one of these mental health challenges. An HBC mother may plunge into postpartum anxiety just a few weeks after birth, and then, over time, she may find that a memory of a particular moment during the birth keeps infiltrating her daily thoughts and exacerbating her struggle with anxiety.

Midwives and doulas are often the only healthcare providers to check in on HBC mothers' mental and emotional health in the days and weeks after birth. They can anticipate that all postpartum women, but particularly HBC women, are at risk for any combination of mental health disorders, and they can routinely screen them for both birth-related PTSD and PMADs. Because the layering of postpartum mood and anxiety disorders, along with PTSD, can make diagnosis more complicated, midwives must ensure that the referrals they give women are for mental health professionals experienced in working with postpartum mothers.

Combined with exhaustion, healing from a surgical birth, caring for a new-born, and partners who may not know how to support them, it is no wonder mothers delay seeking help. Some women are also ashamed to admit that they are struggling or they worry that their child will be taken away if they report to their healthcare provider concerning symptoms such as manic and/or suicidal thoughts.

Recall Julie's traumatic HBC described earlier in this chapter where her midwife discovered her baby was breech during labor. Four months after her birth, Julie took her badly injured dog to the vet. After she carried her dog into the examination room and lay him on the table, the veterinary staff crowded around him and Julie was unable to touch and comfort him. In that moment, Julie's mind flashed back to her own birth and the experience of unfamiliar nurses and doctors crowding around her, performing procedures without her consent, and her feelings of isolation and terror. In the veterinarian's office, Julie began to shake uncontrollably, and she re-experienced the painful raw memories. The next several months brought a heightened sense of anxiety for Julie as she often found herself immersed in the memories and sensations of that moment in the hospital room and in the hallway en route to the operating room. She struggled to process the birth and find resolution, hoping that her grief would dissipate, but instead she would lay awake at night, unable to sleep. Although the term *PTSD* never crossed her mind, Julie knew that her persistent, intrusive memories from the birth were preventing her from enjoying her daily life with her family.

In our interview with birth expert Penny Simkin, she shared three experiences that can occur during labor and birth, which can lead to postpartum PTSD: emotional or physical trauma, fear for self and/or the baby, and feelings of helplessness, loss of control, and being alone.

(For full diagnostic criteria for post-traumatic stress disorder, refer to the Diagnostic and Statistical Manual of Mental Disorders, Fifth Edition [DSM-5].)

For a woman who has a homebirth cesarean, it is common for her to experience birth trauma, and she may then experience PTSD. Birth professionals need to be aware of the potential for HBC trauma and check in with clients throughout their postpartum care about their mental health status, screening them at each visit.

Midwives and doulas often rely on their intuition and the close bond with their clients in order to guess whether a new mother is suffering from a mood and anxiety disorder or PTSD. But mothers may not exhibit obvious outward signs or may mask these signs to maintain the approval of the birth team. Midwives and doulas typically have little to no formal training in evaluating for psychological disorders, and treatment is outside their scope of care. However, midwives and doulas can identify and build relationships with mental health professionals in their communities and readily refer clients who need further assessment and treatment. Birth professionals must also be familiar with local and national phone and online resources for supporting mothers who experienced birth trauma and hand those resources out prenatally. (See Appendix C, Resources for HBC Mothers and Families.)

> How did I go through PTSD with nobody recognizing it? I would sit on my couch all day not going to the bathroom or eating. I would nurse the baby, watch TV, and wait for my husband to get home. Then I would pee, eat a peanut butter sandwich, and never leave the house. That's not normal, but it was normal for me. No one saw the signs or did anything about it.
> —ALEXIS (2011/HBC, MIDWESTERN U.S.)

> With any PTSD, current traumas are triggering old traumas that trigger traumas before them. I had experiences as a young adult and child, situations where I felt trapped. And being in the hospital was like that. It brought up trauma from childhood where I felt like I was being controlled and threatened and there was no way out.
> —BETH (2009/HBC, WESTERN U.S.)

Partners, who are suffering their own psychological and emotional fallout from a homebirth cesarean, may be unequipped to understand and support the mother's mental health concerns. They might see a mother who is acting unlike her former self but have a hard time teasing apart her fatigue and physical healing from a threat to her emotional wellbeing. If the partner has returned to work, he may not notice the often subtle signs of PTSD or he may feel that the experience is in the past and not realize the significant present impact on the birth mother.

With my physical recovery, he was supportive until I started looking better. Then he thought everything was okay and I was healed. Later he just didn't know how to handle a wife who had PTSD. I still don't think he fully gets it.
—CHRISTINE (2012/HBC, WESTERN U.S.)

Triggers

If a mother experiences birth trauma, everything from the birth environment can become coded into her experience and become a trigger later. Common triggers mentioned by the HBC community are hospitals, friends who have out-of-hospital births, recessed lights, dentist appointments, specific foods, songs, birth movies, natural childbirth promotion, and driving at night. Some triggers are obvious in their cause; others are more subtle.

Not only did a woman suffer the effects of the stress response during her birth, but her brain deeply implanted this trauma in her long-term memory. This trauma may later bubble to the surface through flashbacks, nightmares, or recurrent thoughts of a pinpoint moment during the event. When she is removed from the perceived danger, her primal brain registers a trigger, potentially many years later, such as the harsh overhead lighting in her dentist's treatment room, and she plunges back into the trauma of her homebirth cesarean.

This re-experiencing of the stress response during her visit to the dentist is an adaptation to protect her from a situation that presented grave danger in the past, and thus it works to help her avoid that type of danger in the future. In reality, though, she finds this disturbing trigger to be a reminder that the trauma is deep and not merely a bad memory. She might also worry that she will never heal from her birth, or she may suffer feelings of isolation and abandonment once again.

Two years after my birth, my dog had surgery that left him urinating blood during recovery. Seeing his bloody chucks pads on the bathroom floor reminded me of my HBC and brought me to tears hourly. I couldn't look at him without sobbing. My scar even started hurting.
—ANN (2011/HBC, MIDWESTERN U.S.)

*When I think about the events at the hospital, I begin to shake. I can feel the fear
all over again. The pain of the cervical check performed on me by a pumped-up
ER doc who ignored my plea to be gentle is still vivid. Bright lights make my heart
pound as I go straight back to the operating room with my arms strapped down.*
—MELYNDA (2004/HOSPITAL BIRTH, 2007/VBAC TRANSPORT, 2010/HBC, 2013/VBAC
TRANSPORT; SOUTHERN U.S)

Scot Nichols explains that when a person returns to the location of the
traumatic event or something activates a memory of the trauma, the body
is triggered. This triggering can have any number of physical responses
including shaking, shivering, blood flow changes, and alterations in the
perception of the room and people. "That's the body telling you that you
haven't fully returned to safety from the traumatic event," says Nichols.
"Your body is attempting to re-create safety by putting itself back into the
stress response to help you go through the event again, so that this time
you have a successful outcome. The body will recreate triggers repeatedly
because it is literally stuck in the stress response."

A mother may be triggered when visiting the same hospital she was transported to. Her rational brain knows that she is safe as a visitor, yet her
primitive brain, responsible for the stress response, is causing her blood
pressure and heart rate to increase. She breaks out in a cold sweat and feels
afraid. Because the mother knew ahead of time that she would be seeing a
friend who is hospitalized, she prepared for this trigger. She actively mod-
erates her breathing and reminds herself repeatedly that she is not in danger. She cautiously navigates the hospital hallways and finds her friend's
room. This is a casual, unhurried visit, and the HBC mother is able to observe the activity of the hospital staff objectively. As she realizes that no
one is actually going to harm her, her body eases out of the stress response,
allowing her nervous system to potentially lessen the grip of the hospital as
a trigger. The next time she visits the hospital, her stress response may be
reduced, the trigger losing its hold.

I was triggered while visiting the same hospital where I birthed, and my body went into a "react to threat" mode. When I left the hospital, I began running. I ran out of the lobby and just kept running because that was what my body wanted to do. The words coming out of my mouth as I ran were, "Give me back my baby. I'm taking my baby and leaving." Something definitely shifted in the energy patterns of my body and psyche after that. I felt significantly lighter and calmer.
—RACHEL (2009/HBC, WESTERN U.S.)

When a new mother is able to begin the work of processing her trauma by releasing her stored energy, either on her own or with the help of a therapist, she may be able to look ahead to life as a mother who has overcome devastating obstacles.

The remarkable nature of the human brain allows birthing women to persevere through intense physical and emotional challenges. Sometimes, though, these survival mechanisms have such an impact on the new mother that she is at a disadvantage in her healing process, leaving her ill-equipped to begin the journey of motherhood. With a better understanding of how to stay connected to a woman through her labor, surgical birth, and postpartum time, birth professionals have the opportunity to care not only for her physical needs but can also monitor and enhance the emotional well-being of a woman who has a homebirth cesarean.

Birth Professionals' Quick Guide to Trauma

- Routinely discuss early in prenatal care the client's risk factors for traumatic birth and explain the relevance to HBC.

- Provide women with opportunities to privately discuss sensitive health history information during a solo appointment.

- Screen all mothers for perinatal mood and anxiety disorders and birth-related PTSD. (See Appendix E, Screening Tools.)

- Supply referrals for therapy or counseling, encourage women to work through issues that might affect birth, and keep an open dialogue with clients about their progress.

- Use the four points of centering (connect, touch, ask, and narrate) to stay connected to women throughout the birth process.

- Remember that any woman experiencing an HBC may be traumatized by her experience, and ask about her perceptions and feelings throughout the process and afterward.

Chapter 4

From home to the netherworld

I checked in with myself and my baby and the answer was no, I didn't want my midwives to break my water; but I was in such despair that I said yes. Looking back, I see this decision as the moment I stopped listening to myself.

I didn't voice it at the time, but one of the thoughts I had was that I wanted a cesarean. I was born by cesarean myself, and although I didn't want that for my own child's birth, I couldn't stop the idea from coming. I was ashamed even to have that thought and was afraid that saying "cesarean" out loud would make it even more likely to happen. So I said I wanted to transport for pain relief. I thought I would still be able to have a vaginal birth.

My midwives didn't talk to me about why I wanted to go to the hospital. They never asked what I thought was actually going to happen once we got there. No one explained what I might experience. They left the transport decision up to me, but I had been in labor for days and wasn't in a state to make decisions. Where were my midwives telling me I was doing great, that there was nothing wrong, and that we didn't need to go to the hospital?

After I made the decision to transport, I felt like my husband checked out and gave up. The connection we had built during labor was lost. I talk about this with care because I love him so much, but after I decided to transport, he wasn't able to be there for me in the ways that I needed. I think he was in disbelief. He kept saying, "Are we really doing this?" even as he ran around packing a bag.

As soon as I got to the hospital, I felt like it was game-over. I wasn't connected to my baby anymore and felt completely at the mercy of what other people were going to do to me. It was like we went to sleep in laborland and woke up in this netherworld.

My midwives were both engaged with me until the epidural. Then, from what I recall, they emotionally disappeared. I remember them sitting across the room watching me. But I have no memory of them ever talking to me about what I was experiencing during the entire day I labored at the hospital. They

relinquished my care to the hospital staff and were no longer advocating for
me or helping me advocate for myself. I felt like my midwives were witnessing,
rather than supporting. I had to make all the choices, interface with the staff,
and do everything myself.
—RACHEL (2009/HBC, WESTERN U.S.)

After months of anticipation, labor begins. Homebirth supplies are organized in boxes, bags, and small stacks. The mother and her partner try to
rest, quietly enjoying their time together, giddy as they anticipate welcoming their new baby. Hours or days later, the mother has climbed in and out
of the birth tub, her contractions are exhausting, her mouth is dry, and
her shoulders are tense from exertion. Her partner supports her quiver-
ing body, forgetting his own hunger and fatigue. His knees hurt after long
contact with the hard floor, and his upper body is sore from the effort of
providing counter pressure on the mother's sacrum.

Once the decision to transport to the hospital is made, not only does the
landscape of labor change, but, in a moment's time, nine-plus months of
relationship-based midwifery care is drastically replaced by impersonal hospital triage. In this chapter, we traverse the loss of the homebirth
dream and the need for the birth team to continue their compassionate
and knowledgeable support in the hospital. Midwives and doulas can use
the techniques described here to provide physical, emotional, and spiritual
sustenance to the mother and her family.

The transport conversation

Sometimes a laboring woman senses a need for change to help birth her
baby, and understands the hospital might be in her future. Until someone
else broaches the topic of transport, she is often reluctant to articulate what
she already knows, for fear of saying it out loud or disappointing herself
and her birth team.

I needed to transport for a while, but I couldn't get the words out because it
wasn't what I wanted. My midwife told me that the decision had to be 100
percent true to me, in my heart, and I had to accept the outcomes. I'm always
going to wonder: could I have stayed home, and would everything have been
fine? I won't ever know if I made the right choice, and that gets heavy.
—BRANDY (2011/HBC, MIDWESTERN U.S.)

If a midwife or doula suspects that a mother might need to transport, she can begin the conversation in a way that encourages the mother to articulate her perception of the situation. Asking questions such as, "What's going on in your mind right now?" or, "Are you thinking about anything?" gives the mother an opportunity to be heard. Voicing her concerns or fears makes them less threatening, and allows a mother to feel more connected to her birth team. Sometimes she wants to share her insight about the labor; she just needs a prompt.

Midwife Laura Erickson begins the conversation with the mother and her partner as soon as she sees the potential need to transport. Erickson explains what she is observing, clinically and emotionally. She may list factors contributing to the possibility of transport: the mother is exhausted, frustrated, not urinating, the baby is not descending, etc. Narrating the laboring woman's situation creates an opening for the mother to speak, and medically justifies the possible need for transport.

Erickson also finds it helpful to let the mother know, in a non-emergent situation, that she doesn't have to leave for the hospital at once. She reassures her about the immediate health of the baby and acknowledges that the mother is struggling. "I often share that I know labor has been really hard for her," she says. "I tell her it's reasonable and kind to get relief at the hospital. Whatever the situation is, I give her as much detail and support as possible."

> It was the pain of long contractions and the onset of night that terrified me and made me want to go to the hospital, even though I said I could labor at home one more night. After an agonizing contraction, one of my midwives said it was okay to get pain relief, that I didn't have to suffer. Her words allowed me to feel like it was okay to leave home.
> —Ann (2011/HBC, Midwestern U.S.)

> After 40 hours of labor, I really felt like I had given everything I had. When discussing transport, the assistant midwife said, "You don't look like you're enjoying yourself. I want you to know that you don't have to do this. We can find another option. Some part of you should be enjoying yourself." That permission to go to the hospital was such a gift.
> —Alissa (2011/HBC, Western U.S.)

When introducing the possibility of non-emergent transport to a family, birth expert and midwife Mary Jackson strives to "communicate in such a way that we are all making the transport decision together." Like Erickson, Jackson empowers her clients by providing detailed information. "I look at their chart and let them know the time factor," she explains. "I tell them the details of their situation and name all the things that we've tried. Then I talk with the family about options they might want to do at home before we have another transport conversation. When they know that they've tried everything to move labor along safely, it's a lot easier to make the transition to the hospital."

Jackson also speaks directly to the baby, letting him or her know that she's considering a hospital transport. "If you want to be born at home, then we have another hour to see if you can give us a sign of progress," she might say. "I know that you know what to do, and it may be that you want to be born in the hospital. If that's the case, then if there's no progress in an hour, I'll take that as a sign that it's time for us to go." Jackson's willingness to include the baby in the transport decision has a positive impact on the parents' state of mind, reassuring them that everyone in this situation still has a choice.

Making active decisions in labor

Like Rachel, whose story opens this chapter, a woman in the full throes of labor may feel desperate and scared, unable to focus on making an informed, active decision to leave home. In Rachel's case, a combination of exhaustion, memories of her own birth, and unspoken fears precipitated her decision to transport.

In these laboring moments, the mother is engaging the primitive parts of her brain, which are focused on survival rather than strategic decision-making. Outward signs of the mother plunging into the stress response won't be obvious in every situation, but may include a look of panic, darting eyes, fearful, tense, or guarded body language, and an inability to articulate basic needs and to communicate with others.

To guide the mother out of her mounting panic and into active decision-making about transport, the birth team can use the four points of centering: connect, touch, ask, and narrate, introduced in Chapter 3. "I hear that you're scared about going to the hospital," the midwife or doula might say. "I'm right here, supporting you as we make that decision together. Let's take three minutes to talk about what going to the hospital really means. Then you can check in with yourself and your baby. Would that be okay?" The mother may have fewer questions and regrets about her decision to transport if she remembers it as an informed choice she discussed with her birth team.

> With my first, I made the decision to transport, but I didn't have a choice. I was exhausted and my body was done. But with my second, I got to make an active decision. We had a solid plan that we made prenatally, we had a good birth team, and I was clear about my options. These things made the difference between a traumatic and a healing homebirth cesarean.
> —Korin (2006, 2012/HBC; Western U.S.)

Leaving home

Trisha and her partner Carla had excitedly planned a homebirth for their first child. Trisha labored for two days before her contractions became inefficient and spread out. With the aid of their birth team, Trisha made the active decision to transport. Carla tried to adjust to this sudden change of plans as she scrambled around the house looking for a duffel bag, clothes, a toothbrush, and her phone charger. She was worried about Trisha and their baby, but she felt like she needed to get things ready for the transport rather than sit with Trisha through her contractions. Carla was trying to hold herself together for her family while she felt her own mental ability slipping away.

When Carla turned on the overhead light, the room that had been dark for the last 50 hours, was suddenly flooded with disconcerting brightness. The family dog, who had been silent during the long labor, began pacing and whining at the sudden chaos. One midwife was on the phone making arrangements with the hospital, the student midwife was hunting for the baby's first outfit, and the doula was packing the car. Left alone in her bedroom, this abandonment was one of the most traumatic parts of Trisha's HBC, a reality shared by many HBC mothers.

> Once the decision was made, everyone was racing around, working to get out of the house. My husband was rushing to pack a bag, trying to follow a list our doula gave him. Someone asked about the dog, and because everyone was

busy, I had to call our friends to get him while I was going through the worst moments of my life. I was sleep-deprived and started having crazy thoughts about why my baby didn't want to meet me. I hated myself and felt selfish and wretched. During that time alone, I decided I was a waste of a person who couldn't do a damn thing right.
—ANN (2011/HBC, MIDWESTERN U.S.)

We started this journey at 11:45 Friday evening. At 6 a.m. Sunday we made the decision to transport. With that decision, everyone flew into action—Gary and our doula rushed around packing a bag, I got dressed between contractions, our midwife's assistant gathered their supplies and got the bedroom back in order for our eventual return home. Our midwife tried to put things in perspective when our urgency and anxiety grew as we realized that this was not what we planned and that things were about to change.
—LEAH (2012/HBC, WESTERN U.S.)

As the birth team disperses to expedite leaving home, laboring women like Trisha, Ann, and Leah are often left to manage contractions on their own. While her support team is busy attending to the necessary tasks that must be accomplished before everyone can leave, a mother may no longer be sure who is helping her, and may perceive this change of focus as desertion. Now, more than ever, she needs continued attention and support. If she is in the stress response, she will experience a rise in blood pressure, and blood flow to her uterus will dramatically slow as her nervous system launches into survival mode. These and other physiological changes may result in a racing heartbeat and unbearable contractions. Midwives and doulas might notice that a mother begins pacing and taking shallow, panicky breaths. Instead of breathing through contractions, her vocalizations may change to a higher, shriller pitch, and her whole body will tense with every contraction.

To facilitate a non-emergent transport while still providing emotional care to the mother, it's important for the midwife or doula to gather everyone involved, including the mother, and clarify roles. Who is responsible for the immediate tasks at hand? Who will stay with the mother and provide continuous support? The birth team can ask the mother open-ended questions, offering her the opportunity to share her concerns. "Are you emotionally ready to leave home? What can we do to help you? Is there anything you want to try before leaving?" This huddle offers a moment of re-connection before the drive to the hospital and a plan to guide the transport.

As part of this birth team huddle, the family's highest intention for birth can also be acknowledged. Wanting an out-of-hospital birth goes deeper than the desire to have a baby at a specific location. A plan for a homebirth is often a way to meet the family's needs for privacy, autonomy, respect, lack of interventions, or the avoidance of judgment by strangers. Midwives and doulas are usually aware of a family's intentions, and during a transport it is their job to reassure the family that they will stay with the mother, help her advocate for herself, and try to maintain her intentions wherever possible, despite the change of setting.

Perhaps a couple's decision to birth outside of the hospital is linked to their personal need for privacy. Reflecting on that intention, their midwife or doula can remind the mother that although she is changing her birthing setting, that goal remains the same. She can explain how the birth team will work to create privacy for her at the hospital, though it will look different than privacy at home—advocating for alone time before and after decisions and whenever she needs moments to reconnect with her partner, herself, and her baby. Aware that her birth team understands and is committed to her intention, the mother might feel more ready to accept the transport.

Whenever possible, the midwife can give the couple time alone together before leaving home or the birth center, even for just a few minutes. They are likely to be in some degree of distress at this point; but here, too, the birth team can provide guidance, suggesting that they take time to hug each other and to grieve this change in plans. The midwife or doula can prompt the mother to check in with her baby, remind the partner to remain focused and connected to the mother, and urge them both to carry this bond throughout the hospital experience.

Even in an emergency transport, there are ways to decrease the stress for the family. The midwife, when calling 911, can clarify the level of urgency and request that the paramedics quietly approach the home or birth center. There is also a brief window of time before the ambulance arrives when the midwife or doula can help the mother dress and talk about what to expect, and about the barrage of decisions they will need to make. The midwife can tell the mother that, if possible, she will stay with her in the ambulance or will meet her at the hospital. She can remind the mother that once at the hospital, her role as midwife will change, and that the mother and her partner will have to assert their needs and choices once they get there.

Before leaving home, the birth team can facilitate a moment of closure for the transporting family. This could be a brief ritual: a minute of silence for the labor and the bond they shared at home, a verbal acknowledgement of the sacredness of their time, a prayer, or flowers left at the threshold of the front door.

Partners transporting

Laura Erickson understands that part of her job as a midwife is to help partners, and she uses the same approach with them that she uses with laboring mothers. "I know you've been up for two nights," she might say to a partner. "You must be getting tired. Your mom keeps calling on the phone, and that can be frustrating." Gently, Erickson guides the tired partner, makes sure she eats, helps her pack, even reminds her to use the bathroom before they leave. "These moments with the partner are vital," she says, "The partner's attitude can influence the mama's."

> Leaving home was mostly a huge relief, as the labor had lasted longer than I could have imagined. I knew that the doctors would be able to help us at the hospital in ways that the midwives couldn't.
> —ALEX, PARTNER OF CARRIE (2011/HBC, WESTERN U.S.)

> The change was so black and white, and I was in shock that we were leaving, but I trusted what Alissa needed for her body. My mind was racing to remember all the things to watch out for at the hospital while we scrambled to pack the essentials. Our birth team made sandwiches, which was a life saver. I was so relieved that our midwives were driving us to the hospital. I can't even imagine having to find my way there under those conditions.
> —COBALT, PARTNER OF ALISSA (2012/HBC, WESTERN U.S.)

The car ride

Many women we interviewed found it comforting to have their midwife or doula ride with them to the hospital. Their presence in the car helped maintain continuity of care and reassured them, especially while their partners were focused on driving. After continuous care during labor, the prospect of being without the support of the birth team at this dark hour is daunting. The simple act of riding in the car with the mother can both provide comfort and help the birth team bridge the homebirth energy from home to the hospital.

Gail Tully, founder of Spinning Babies, an optimal fetal positioning technique, points out that even if a woman actively chooses to leave home under non-emergent circumstances, she or her partner may still think that the baby is in serious danger. A mother is not thinking rationally so as to appreciate the clinical factors at hand. "By transporting, midwives are telling moms that they can't help them at home anymore," Tully says. "Even if the midwives don't perceive the mother or baby to be in a critical situation, the laboring woman might see the transport as a life or death scenario. And that's traumatic for anyone to go through."

> I was separated from my midwife in the car and it was terrifying for me. I was scared, I was sad, I felt like a failure. No one was there to tell me that things were safe.
> —Ashley (2011/HBC, Southern U.S.)

> I should not have been driving after being awake for three days. I was manic and behind the wheel of a car, alone with my laboring wife who had meconium pouring from her vagina. Then I was following a midwife who was only 80% sure where she was going.
> —Dave, partner of Courtney (2011/HBC, Western U.S.)

> As the driver, I felt it was essential to have our midwife with us in the car so someone could support Jo. My anxiety was reduced knowing that the midwife was taking care of her, talking to her, and encouraging her. Since the hospital was not part of our plan, we were already highly stressed and feeling ill-prepared, so her presence was crucial to helping me be calm and centered.
> —Cath, partner of Jo, (2012/HBC, Western U.S.)

Logistical reasons may prevent the midwife or doula from accompanying the mother in the car. In this situation, the midwife can offer phone support to the family during the drive through speaker phone contact.

Birth team support in the hospital

The one-on-one support must continue from home to car to the hospital, but if the midwife is unable to accompany the family, it is vital that she clearly explain her reasons to the mother. It is equally important to tell the mother exactly who will be supporting her instead. The midwife can also make it clear that she intends to resume care for the family as soon as possible. This direct communication will reassure the mother that her midwife is not abandoning her because she is transporting and "failing" at her homebirth.

When the birth team includes a midwife and a student midwife, unless the mother has a stronger connection with the apprentice, the primary midwife must go to the hospital with the family. An apprentice typically has limited experience supporting a mother, and will be less familiar with the hospital staff and interventions. In addition, sending only the apprentice on a transport may inadvertently communicate the message that because the mother cannot birth at home, she does not deserve the care of her full birth team.

If labor has been long and the birth team is tired, they have several options for maintaining continuous support of the family. The birth team can offer choices to the family, such as the least tired midwife going to the hospital while another stays to clean the home and rest. Alternatively, the entire team can go to the hospital and take shifts resting, ready to support the mother as needed. If only one midwife is attending the birth, she can obtain the mother's consent to call a backup midwife to meet them at the hospital. No matter which option is chosen, the primary midwife can communicate the plan to the mother, letting her know how her birth team will support her while getting the rest they need.

> I wait until my client is sleeping, and then try to get some sleep in the room with her, but I'll wake up during vaginal checks and procedures to provide support and help answer questions she may have. I also bring my student midwife with me and we alternate taking short breaks, sleeping, going for walks, anything that helps us stay alert and present. If mom is asleep or content with us taking a break together, I'll usually pull my student out of the room so she can ask questions in private.
>
> —Amanda Roe, naturopathic midwife, Western U.S.

Predators everywhere

The move from home to hospital is usually a negative physical, emotional, and psychological change for the mother. In an attempt to protect herself and her baby, she instinctually builds mental and energetic barriers against unfamiliar hospital protocols, unwanted interventions, and the presence of strangers. She may withdraw, argue with nurses and doctors, or lose connection with her baby as she ceases engaging with others as a way to protect her psyche.

One of the effects of the instinctual stress response is that the reptilian brain loses its ability to understand nuances in body language and communication. As a result, the mother identifies everything in her environment as a threat and she may feel unsure if her birth team or hospital staff is "on her side." The mother may perceive that a tired doula is angry with her or think her partner is annoyed when he is merely confused by what is happening.

When the depleting nature of labor is layered with the physiologic effects of the stress response, women are unable to understand the expressions of those around them or maintain open communication. In this illustration, the laboring mother is depicted as a frightened alligator, which represents her primitive reptilian brain. She is surrounded by nurses and doctors whom she perceives as foreign, out of place, and threatening to her and her baby's safety.

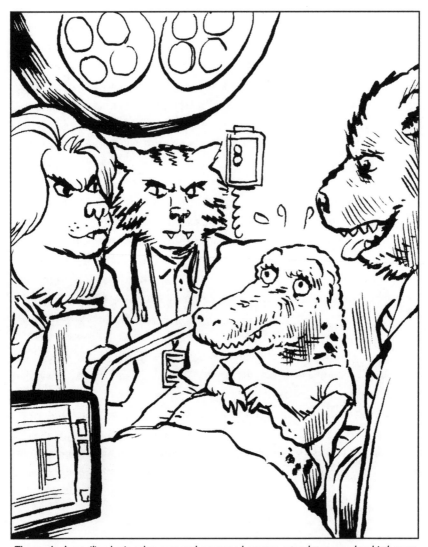

The mother's reptilian brain takes over and everyone becomes a predator, even her birth team.

Reklaw, 2013

When a mother senses her environment as threatening, it can be impossible for her to ask for help. Women's health physical therapist Tami Lynn Kent says that HBC women in her practice often report wanting more support from their midwives than they received. "Even if their midwife is present and sitting across the hospital room," Kent explains, "a laboring mom might be unable to make verbal requests of them. The more a mama gets into the fatigue and longevity of labor, the harder it gets for her to ask for the support she needs."

For their part, once in the hospital environment, the birth team may find it more difficult to assess the mother's needs, even if they have maintained a steady physical and emotional connection with her. This may be due in part to the mother's protective barriers or the birth team's own comfort level in the hospital.

Midwife Mary Jackson likes to check in on a laboring mother if she has been focused inwardly for some time. "I softly ask how she is feeling. I watch her breathing patterns, because they often signal something different from her words. I look for a contrast between her body freezing in rigidity and a calm stillness that connotes fluidity and acceptance." Perhaps the hospital environment has triggered flashbacks to previous trauma or even to memories of her own birth. "If I find that she is internally panicking, I ask the mother to open her eyes and look around the room and see who is with her and where she is," Jackson explains. "I ask her to assess her safety with her eyes open, because closing her eyes can amplify a past experience and not allow her to connect to what is occurring in the moment."

Glimpses from the hospital

> We talked to our midwives before every decision. It was another 30 hours in the hospital before the actual cesarean, and they were there the entire time. They said I did a good job as I was laboring and strapped to the bed. They told me that I was doing everything I could, that I couldn't do anything differently, and that I was making the right choice about every decision I made. They were amazing.
> —LIBBY (2011/HBC, 2013/VBAC TRANSPORT; MIDWESTERN U.S.)

> At the least, I wanted my midwife to bring things to my attention in the hospital and say, "Hey, you might want to think about this" or, "Remember what we talked about regarding X intervention?" That didn't happen. With every question that came up, I had to ask her, "What do you think?" She wouldn't speak up on her own. That's when the feelings of abandonment and resentment started. At around 37 weeks, I'd asked her to look over the hospital birth plan I was writing. She pointed to herself and said, "It's not necessary—if we transfer, I'm your birth plan." But she wasn't. She wasn't at all.
> —LEAH (2012/HBC, WESTERN U.S.)

My midwife said she was not going to the hospital because she was a home-birth midwife and had another client in labor.
—CARA (2005, 2007/HB, 2008/HBC; WESTERN U.S.)

Our midwife ditched us. She said, "I know you really want your sister and husband there, and there's really no official task for me at the hospital, so I'm just not going." She didn't ask us; it wasn't a question.
—LIZ (2008/HBC, NORTHEASTERN U.S.)

Prenatally, our midwife said she would stay and support us at the hospital. I even paid an additional upfront fee for her to continue care during a transport. It wasn't until we got to the hospital that she said she was leaving to get some sleep and that we should call her when I was pushing. I felt scared not having her there, but there was also a part of me that was trying to take care of her because I knew she was tired. When my husband called her, she said she couldn't come because she was heading to another birth. I felt abandoned and resentful because she was going to a "normal" birth. At that point, I wasn't in a state to advocate for myself, and my midwife didn't offer to send any of our other three midwives to the hospital.
—DANA (2012/HBC, WESTERN U.S.)

Our midwives spoke up for our needs without hesitation. They knew what we wanted from the beginning, and they had their heads on straight at the hospital. They were our voices when we couldn't speak. I appreciate how much they stepped in and made it clear to the staff what we wanted.
—JAKE, PARTNER OF CAROL (2012/HBC, WESTERN U.S.)

Rachel experienced a profound disconnection from her midwives at the hospital that she shared with us in this written piece:

I felt like the midwives were sitting at a great distance across the hospital room. They had all the energy of people at a funeral or a deathbed. Gone were the encouragements, the focus, the reminders. No touch was offered. There was a vast divide between the hospital bed and them in their stiff chairs. Maybe they were trying to create a supportive circle by giving my husband and me space to be together, but it felt like they had abandoned us. I gave up by going to the hospital, and now they had given up on me. They were the mirror of my own defeat.

I feel like my midwives were scared by my fears and needed to make them go away. But my fears wouldn't go away without being looked at. Where was the grounded, knowing midwife, asking, "What are you afraid of? Speak it out loud so we can hold it to the light and transform it." No one reminded me, at my darkest hour, of my higher intention. No one said, "Yes, you feel scared. Yes, you feel like you are going to die."

The faces of my midwives showed defeat, guilt, and hopelessness. I looked across the hospital room for something, and that's what I was met with: It's already happened. Your baby is already sliced from you. We are watching it happen and can do nothing to stop it.

Collaboration with hospital staff

The way the birth team interacts with the mother and the hospital staff directly impacts the mother's perception of her baby's safety, and that of her own. Midwives and doulas can make it a point to show collaboration and cooperation with hospital personnel. Midwives can ask the nurses and OB/GYN to partner with her in making the family's experience as smooth as possible. Midwife Lori Cohen says:

> I try to get them on our team from the outset and also make it a point to show my gratitude for their willingness to help and care for my clients. This has been a fantastic way of gently guiding doctors to care for women compassionately, since I have just thanked them in advance for doing so. I also tell them that I think the mom will really need me to support her, and I give the OB permission to tell me how I can be helpful. It might come across to the mother as "being on the doctor's side," but it can help the staff to know that I acknowledge their situation and will be flexible in working with them, while still supporting my client.

There is a fine line between showing cooperation with staff and "taking their side," which can be perceived by the reptilian brain as ganging up on the mother to coerce her to agree to a cesarean. However, partnering with the hospital staff while also advocating for the mother and supporting her needs helps her both in the moment and later, when she is processing her birth.

The partner in the hospital

The sense of abandonment a mother often feels in the hospital is heightened if there are emotional or physical barriers between her and her partner. From a partner's perspective, there are many roadblocks to staying connected with the mother. In addition to an IV pole, bed rails, and machines, partners are also aware that they are no longer witnessing the spontaneous nature of labor. They may feel nervous about the protocol-driven, highly technological hospital experience that no longer involves them. Their fatigue, fears, self-blame, and personal discomfort all threaten to break down their ability to care for the mother. Partners are also reacting to the mother's inability to communicate, so when the reptilian brain interprets that their partner is angry, mothers may stop looking to their partners for support. The partner then sees that the mother is rebuffing their attempts at connection with her, and they begin to shut down. If a partner senses the mother doesn't want him around, he may begin withdrawing support.

From the hospital's perspective, the medical team is solely focused on the mother's and baby's health, and typically aren't aware of the nature of the mother's relationship with her partner, nor do they have time to explore this during the labor and birth. As a result, partners can feel extraneous and shut out from the birth of their child.

> I felt like a little kid in an adult setting where people didn't want to hear from me until they were ready. Everyone was a worker bee doing their one job to make the birth machine work. The closer I tried to be to Courtney, the more in the way I was of everyone else. I was wrapped in anxiety and disorientation. There were clipboards, blaring lights, and no one was tender to my wife. No one ever held space for Courtney.
> —DAVE, PARTNER OF COURTNEY (2011/HBC, WESTERN U.S.)

> I hated the hospital; it was terrifying. I would have gone crazy had two of the three midwives not gone with us. Their presence was vital.
> —JIM, PARTNER OF REBECCA (2012/HBC, SOUTHERN U.S.)

> I had to put aside my anger and frustrations to do my best to support and keep a positive focus on Amy.
> —RICK, PARTNER OF AMY (2011/HBC, NORTHEASTERN U.S.)

*The hospital treated us horribly from the moment we arrived. I felt like they
didn't even want us there and that we were an annoyance to them.*
—GARY, PARTNER OF TRISHA (2007/HBC, NORTHEASTERN U.S.)

The birth team can offer their support to partners by asking them questions about their experience: "What's going on for you right now? What
do you think about the doctor wanting to break her water?" Midwives and
doulas can normalize partners' feelings and suggest ways in which they can
care for themselves and the mother. Reminding partners about the family's rights in the hospital and explaining what is happening during interventions is also a way to draw partners out of their protective shell. If the
partner is someone who benefits from having a task, the birth team can be
sure that the partner is guided on how to care for the mother using the four
points of centering—connect, touch, ask, narrate.

Cascade of losing control

"Cesarean begins with the capture of a woman's power," says birth healer and midwife, Sister MorningStar, "long before a knife pierces the skin."
The longer a woman labors in the hospital, the more her options dwindle
because of the imposition of timelines, protocols, and the culture of expediency. For a laboring mother, this can feel like the hospital is trying to take
away her control. In the hospital's point of view, they have a very short window to assess the urgency of the situation, along with the prenatal and labor
care the mother received. Lara Williams, OB/GYN, notes that it is a "huge
responsibility to accept a patient whom you know nothing about and who
is now firmly your medical and legal responsibility."

A mother in the hospital relinquishes control of her labor, her body, her
baby, and now she must contend with numerous interventions. She may
feel unable to stop the train of madness that she perceives her birth is becoming, and she may surrender her decision-making autonomy. Further-
more, hospital staff rarely recognize and acknowledge the mental, spiritual, and emotional pain of a transport. Often they simply see a homebirth
mother who might be difficult to work with because she is protesting interventions. But when hospital personnel do recognize the distress of transport and offer choices in her care whenever possible, the mother can feel
that she maintains her dignity and her right to self-determination.

My nurse spoke to me in the sweetest, most gentle tones and right away gave me compliments about my character and what a good mom I was going to be. As if I couldn't get any luckier, my anesthesiologist went above and beyond in his effort to befriend me. I feel indebted to the hospital staff for showing me so much love and kindness.
—Robyn (2012/HBC, Western U.S.)

With the guidance of her birth team, a mother can focus on her highest intention for the birth, and she can clarify and communicate her non-negotiables. For example, if she asserts her choice for no cervical checks without consent, being in the hospital can feel less like giving in, since her self-determination and power to negotiate for her needs are maintained. A laboring woman needs her partner and her birth team to help her advocate for her choices. Her midwife and doula can guide her as she asserts her right to respect, privacy, and safety. HBC mother Ann says, "I've wondered so many times why my midwives or doula didn't remind me that I could have said no to all these strangers giving me rough vaginal exams. No one said that to me, and I really wish they had." (See Appendix A, Plan C for more information about non-negotiables.)

It would have made a huge difference if my midwives had said, "This is our recommendation at this point in time." They could have asked, "Would you like some time alone for just you and your baby, to check in? Let's talk about what this intervention means and what you can do." To have an overt choice-point again, rather than this cascade of losing control, is huge. How can I be empowered now? And now? And now?
—Rachel (2009/HBC, Western U.S.)

Mothers are often less traumatized if they feel included in decision-making, so I encourage birth teams to find a way to ask doctors and nurses some version of the following: "Can you make sure this mother feels that she is fully participating in making this decision?"
—Ananda Lowe, doula and author, Northeastern U.S.

A woman moving toward surgical birth needs to know that she did everything within her capacity to make choices that were right for her and her baby. If this doesn't happen, she may feel like a victim, and that she lacked autonomy during her birth. Choice is fundamental to her well-being and mental health, and choice will profoundly impact the way she remembers her birth experience, not only in the days and weeks to come, but in the memories she will carry for a lifetime.

Birth Professionals' Quick Guide to Transport

- Use the four points of centering—connect, touch, ask, narrate—throughout labor.

- Explain to partners the transport process, ensure their basic needs are met, and show them how to stay connected to the mother and baby.

- Lead a birth team huddle before leaving home.

- Remain present, always telling the mother when you will see her again if you need to be apart.

- Remember that the mother, if she is in the fight-or-flight or the freeze stress response, is seeing everything through the filter of survival and will not be able to communicate her needs.

- Help the mother advocate for her needs, keeping her highest birth intention in mind, and reminding her she has choice-points throughout her labor at the hospital.

Birth Story:
Midwifing the Midwife. The Partner's Perspective

Rick is partner to Samantha, an apprentice homebirth midwife who chose her mentor midwife to provide care during her birth. In this story crafted from Rick's interview seven months after the birth, he shares his anger and resentment.

Samantha would have been a lot better off if she hadn't been treated like a midwife having a baby. I went to most prenatal appointments, but when I wasn't there, I know there were a lot of half-conversations about important subjects because Samantha was so knowledgeable about birth. But a midwifery apprentice is not the same thing as a mom in labor.

When the midwife came to check on her the first time during labor, she assumed Samantha was more dilated than she actually was. The midwife told her she wasn't able to relax and let go enough for labor to keep progressing and it mentally played on Samantha. It became Samantha trying hard to keep labor going by walking and squatting because that is what the midwife expected. Samantha pushed herself too far.

The midwife left to give us space and told me to help Samantha "let go." I was put in charge of everything. But I needed the midwife to be there for us. I didn't want to be in charge, so I called her back.

After about 24 hours of labor, Samantha knew she needed to go to the hospital for more fluids and she initiated the transport conversation. Once at the hospital, the departure point for me with the midwife was when Samantha was in the bathtub trying to calm down because she was so out of it. The midwife made a comment about "needing to do everything we can to prevent a cesarean." Samantha just looked at her and said, "I really don't want you to say that because if I have a cesarean, I don't want to feel bad about it." That was the end of my relationship with the midwife. Who says such a thing in labor?

When Samantha was taken to the operating room to be prepped, I was sobbing buckets. It was an emotional wellspring bubbling out of me and a pretty devastating moment. I ran into the bathroom to call my brother, who is a doctor. I needed a pep talk. He reminded me that when this was over, I would have a baby. It's hard to accept everything in the moment, but between my brother and my father-in-law's support, they kept me from completely falling apart.

In the operating room I had a hard time watching how her body was treated. They were moving her around like a piece of meat. I know that she has a deep relationship with her body and for her to not be able to feel her pelvis or uterus is hard to imagine. Watching that was very traumatic for me.

It is endlessly sad that Samantha didn't get to hold her son first, because she deserved to. I didn't want to be with our baby without her. I wanted to stay with her, but she insisted I go to the warming table. It wasn't what I wanted for her. Samantha was happy that I got to have that special moment, but for me it's tragic.

The one thing that was really hard for Samantha was that the midwife didn't come to visit after the birth. Technically, we didn't need her to come, but Samantha wanted her to check in. She felt abandoned because she needed her for the emotional part of it. We were told prenatally what the postpartum visit schedule would be, and then she didn't even call.

Samantha was the one who got in touch with her first. The midwife told her she thought she had been fired and she chose not to come because of the "vibe she was getting from us." That's what she felt energetically, but Samantha didn't say that she didn't want her. She resumed care with the midwife, but I didn't participate in the visits.

The last time Samantha saw her, she told Samantha I was an angry dad and that my opinion about her care was out of anger. That's really not fair and it's super-manipulative. It caused a lot of trouble for Samantha in terms of her own process and grief resolution. I plan on giving the midwife feedback, but I have not yet been able to because at this point it *would* sound angry. In time, it will happen.

In order to deal with the birth, Samantha and I made a pact that whatever we're feeling, we are going to say it to each other. It's so important to be able to express those hard things instead of worrying about if it's okay to feel a certain way. It's difficult to process having a birth that is so joyous and mixed with a lot of sadness, disappointment, and some regret.

At the end of the day, dads are taught to be the protector and provider, and I accept that role. But in the operating room, I lost the ability to take care of my partner and our baby. It was traumatic for me and I have a lot of feelings about it.

For Samantha, one of the things she took away is that she had some emotional block that didn't allow her body to dilate, basically, that something was wrong with her body. So, I just want her to know that her body is great, because it is great.

Chapter 5

Initiation by scalpel

I thought I was dying. They wheeled the stretcher from the ambulance to the operating table; I had no idea where I was. Everyone was talking at once, wearing masks. I labored at home for 17 hours, and then suddenly I was in an operating room. The doctor told me they were going to put me under for a cesarean, and the thought flashed through my mind that I had been ripped from my home and thrown into a horrible George Orwell novel. I started screaming for my midwife. She appeared, but I couldn't see her mouth moving behind her mask. It felt like an alien abduction. The doctor looked at me and with a thick Russian accent said, "You could give birth vaginally, but your baby will die."

I went into a very dark, deep sleep. I saw the blue sheet go up and thought I would wake up on the other side of that sheet dead. I figured that was what death felt like: a nurse guides you to count backward from 100.

When I woke up, I was in a recovery room. It was quiet; there was a nurse, a beeping machine, and no one else. Everything was calm and I wasn't in pain. I thought my baby was dead because he wasn't with me. I knew what I wanted to ask, but I didn't dare say it out loud. Was my son alive? Was he alone?

They wheeled me into a room and my birth team was there. It was like the Wizard of Oz because it felt like years had passed, yet everyone was exactly the way they were when I left them. Jake carried our son to me.
—CAROL (2012/HBC, WESTERN U.S.)

The birth of Carol's surprise breech baby became an emergency situation, leaving her and her birth team without time to advocate in the operating room. Her experience stands in sharp contrast to Ann's non-emergent birth, during which her birth team was able to negotiate on her behalf:

I woke from a nap to the doctor shaking my arm, saying, "Ready for your cesarean?" I didn't know where I was or what had happened. I couldn't understand anything because I didn't remember we had transported to the hospital.

As they were about to wheel me out of the room, I realized that when the baby was born, my husband was going to have to decide if he should stay with his sobbing, traumatized wife or his new child. That was a rotten decision for him, so I asked for my doula as a second support person.

The doctor kept repeating that there was no room in the OR. My support team was looking at me to stand up to this guy. I'm usually a sassy person, but I was so broken that I couldn't do it. I just shrugged and said I was too tired to fight.

They started wheeling me out and one of my midwives put her hand on the bed. "This conversation hasn't ended. These people have been through a lot. They're exhausted and traumatized, and we need to have a real talk about why they can't have their support person there."

The doctor got mad. "What don't you understand about there being no room in the OR?" The midwife asked if there would be students present. He said there were two. She turned to me and said, "Ann, you have the right to decline the presence of those students. Do you want to decline?" I said I declined, and my doula was allowed in because we made space in the OR.
—ANN (2011/HBC, MIDWESTERN U.S.)

In this chapter, beginning with the cesarean decision, continuing through the surgical birth, and ending in the recovery room, we walk the dark HBC journey with mothers and partners. We explore how to support a mother through a homebirth cesarean and show that her surgical initiation into motherhood is difficult, powerful, and meaningful.

The conscious cesarean decision

The decision to move ahead with a cesarean is based on many factors, including the mother's and baby's health, her emotions and intuition, and the support or pressure from those around her. For some women the decision comes after a period, however brief, of consideration with the full support of their birth team. For families who experienced a pre-labor HBC, the decision to schedule a cesarean may take days or weeks. Unfortunately, the majority of mothers we interviewed said cesarean was not much of a choice at all. It was thrust upon them due to circumstance, lack of support, or urgency.

A decision implies choice and I was given none. The OB wouldn't meet with me and no one explained why a cesarean was the best option. I don't remember knowing when I signed the consent form that I was actually agreeing to a cesarean. How do I own a decision that I don't feel I actually had a choice in?
—JULIA (2002, 2004, 2008/HOSPITAL BIRTH, 2006, 2011/HB, 2013/HBC; CANADA)

Feeling ownership requires having clarity about why a cesarean is preferable and what other options are still available. Asking the doctor specific questions helps the mother understand the medical reasons for a surgical birth. With this awareness, she can explain under what conditions she would consent to a cesarean. She may also feel empowered to try other things to avoid the operating room.

As part of seeking clarity regarding why a cesarean is recommended, some women found it helpful to meet with their surgeon so they could potentially form a connection with the doctor or request another physician. This approach can lessen the stranger aspect of a surgical birth and validate a mother's decision to move forward.

The cesarean was posed as an emergency, but later I realized it was a choice.
—RACHEL (2009/HBC, WESTERN U.S.)

Mothers often feel they only have two choices when a cesarean is offered: they can consent because it's the only option left, or they can refuse because there are still options remaining to try to change the course of the birth. But in reality there is a third choice in which a woman can say, "This isn't what I want, and it's not the only option left, but it feels like the best option right now." Awareness that this third choice exists can potentially lessen the guilt she may carry about her decision to move forward with surgery.

At the moment of the cesarean decision, I told myself, "Beth, you need to be present. Remember that you are choosing this. Remember that you made this decision because you decided it was the right thing to do."
—BETH (2009/HBC, WESTERN U.S.)

In these non-emergent situations, the birth team can ensure that the family has privacy prior to making a final decision. This grants them grieving time, helps them regain connection with each other, allows them to begin considering next steps, and gives them space to formulate questions.

> *One of my biggest regrets is that I didn't realize I could have kicked the hospital staff out of my room and had a moment with my partner, mother, and midwives to come to a decision together. I really would have benefitted from that. Even if everything else would have gone the same way, I could have felt as if I had an actual part in making the decision for the surgery.*
> —Jo (2012/HBC, Western U.S.)

> *My partner and I had a chance to talk about it alone. I knew if I was going to have a cesarean, I wanted to be in control of the situation as much as possible, so I liked the idea of consenting when it wasn't an emergency and I was fully present.*
> —Kim (2001/HBC, Midwestern U.S.)

Midwife Mary Jackson knows that often homebirth mothers prefer to connect with their babies internally to receive knowledge about their health and well-being. To a woman who feels comfortable doing so, Jackson tells her to "go inward and get her own information, because she knows her baby best."

> *I knew something was horribly wrong—my baby was trying to tell me that it wasn't right for him to be born naturally. I was begging for a cesarean but they wanted me to keep pushing. That knowing never left me throughout the surgery.*
> —Anna (2003/hospital birth, 2012/HBC; United Kingdom)

Negotiating before consenting

Once a mother has made a cesarean decision, she needs to advocate for her specific wishes prior to consenting by saying something like, "Yes, I'm ready to have a cesarean if my doula can come into the operating room with me and my partner." This request can open the conversation in a way that maintains her choice and self-determination, which is what homebirth mothers desire.

Often doctor's reasons are not always obvious for doing things against a family's wishes. The reasons for exclusion of a second support person, if given, vary from liability to safety to control. Donald Flynn, MD, an OB anesthesiologist, says that for him, it's a matter of physical space in the operating room. "To do my job as an anesthesiologist with two additional people sitting at mom's head is difficult. The space I have to work in is actually very small. My main function is to make sure mom is safe, but I have to ensure her support person is safe as well. If there is a second person with her, that makes three people I need to be in charge of. I can't do my job effectively if I don't have the space I need, or if I'm distracted by two other people."

If the anesthesiologist doesn't want to allow the second support person due to liability, the mother can mirror back to the doctor that she understands his point of view, saying something like, "I understand that you're worried about extra bodies that could get in the way or be distracting. I know that makes your job harder. But I need that extra support for me to do my job, which is to give birth by cesarean." The mother can also share what she has already given up to get to where she is in this moment, trying to draw upon the doctor's empathy and connection as a human being. Having done this, she needs to know that she will probably have to give up something else in the name of negotiating, like delayed cord clamping. She needs to be clear on her biggest needs and be willing to pick and choose from her Plan C. (See Appendix A, Plan C to help identify needs during a surgical birth.)

If a second person is not allowed in the OR, the mother can request that a nurse specifically act as her emotional support person and advocate during the surgery. The nurse can introduce her to the staff in the operating room, narrate what is happening, and help her stay connected with her partner during the surgery.

> The last time I attended a homebirth cesarean, I was cheek to cheek with the mother in the OR, regulating my breath to help her regulate hers. I was speaking softly and slowly into her ear and holding her shoulder through the entire birth. While she shook and went through panic and terror I was narrating, "Now they are making the first incision, now they are..." and, "I feel your body shaking. I am right here with you. I will stay right here with you."
> —SILKE AKERSON, CPM, WESTERN U.S.

Another negotiation in non-emergent situations is the mother keeping her placenta. Many homebirth mothers want to see their placenta, encapsulate it for medicinal use, or bury it as a memorial. If taking the placenta home is a strong intention for the family, it can also be used as a negotiation tool before consenting. If the doctor agrees to release the placenta to the family, someone can tell the hospital staff in the operating room not to put it in preservatives, and possibly another reminder will need to be given after surgery. If the doctor wants to send the placenta to pathology, the mother can suggest they take a small sample for the lab and leave the remainder with her.

> The first time I wanted to make prints with my placenta and plant it in the garden. For my second, I hired someone to make a tincture. Both times my placenta was sent to pathology without my consent. Not seeing my placentas was devastating. I lost a connection with any physical evidence that my baby had ever been attached to and nourished by me.
> —Stephanie (2008, 2012/HBC; Northeastern U.S.)

Other women we interviewed reported negotiating for immediate skin-to-skin contact after birth and breastfeeding in the operating room. Whatever a mother's highest intention is during a cesarean, her birth team can help her clarify what is most important to her and remain by her side during the negotiation process.

Using the four points of centering: A movie scene

Hospital Room, Labor and Delivery - Night

A bright hospital delivery room. An air of resignation prevails as the family privately decides that cesarean is the only option left. The fetal monitor spits out paper, charting the baby's heart rate. Machines beep. The Partner is silent, hands in pockets, staring at the floor.

The Midwife bends over the hospital bed, her head close to a quiet laboring woman. She places her hand on the mother's thigh and asks, "May I tell you what's about to happen?" The Mother nods her head. The Partner perks up.

Looking with compassion into the Mother's eyes, the Midwife says: "I want you to know that I'm right here, supporting you. If I'm not allowed in the OR, I'll wait for you in this room. When you get to the OR, it's going to be cold and everyone will be wearing masks. The anesthesiologist will be sitting near your head and your Partner will join you before they start the surgery."

The Midwife pauses to allow the information to sink in. The Mother's tears stream down her face. The Partner is now holding her hand.

The Midwife touches the Mother's belly and says to the Baby: "Hi Baby. You are about to meet your Mama. It's different from what we thought would happen and I know you know that already. A doctor will lift you out of your home and it's going to be bright and cold. As soon as possible, you will join your Mama, who loves you very much and can't wait to hold you."

The Midwife looks to the Mother: "What's going on for you right now?"

Between sobs: "I feel sick."

Midwife: "What's making you feel sick?"

Shakes head: "Because they might take my baby away."

Midwife: "Are you okay talking about our Plan C?" The Mother nods. The Midwife begins rubbing the Mother's thigh, and the Partner squats to be at eye level with her.

"I hear that you are scared that you might not be able to hold your baby right after birth. Like we talked about, before consenting to the cesarean, we can negotiate for immediate skin-to-skin contact and that you want to save your placenta. I'll be with you, by your side, as you make those requests." The Midwife notices that the Mother's breathing becomes more rhythmic and sees the Partner squeeze her hand and kisses her forehead.

Midwife: "I know this isn't what you wanted, and I'm sorry it's happening this way. It's okay to grieve that loss." Long pause as her body begins to shake with sobs. The Partner assures her that he will be with her in the operating room, holding her hand. He tells her that she is strong and that he loves her.

The Midwife hugs both Mother and Partner before leaving to give them a few minutes of privacy.

The partner alone

The partner's perception that the mother or baby will be hurt at the hospital can activate her own fight-or-flight or freeze stress response, and affect her ability to connect with and support the laboring mother. Liz Robinson, a hospital nurse midwife, has seen the full spectrum of partners' involvement during homebirth transfers. "By the time people come to us, they are exhausted, and I'm not sure how much they're really hearing me, so I try to give the partners lots of support," says Robinson. "I know how traumatic it has been for them to watch Mom, and they feel responsible for protecting her from what we might do to her. So I just try to love them up."

After the cesarean decision, the partner is separated from the mother while she is prepped for surgery. This creates a sense of helplessness in partners that is "confusing and mostly indescribable," as one father put it.

Midwife Amanda Roe says that from her experience, "Most partners waiting to get called into surgery are shell-shocked. Usually they're just going through the motions. The labor has been hard for them to watch; then the cesarean decision gets made and it all happens so fast. I feel like I lose connection with them after the decision. I don't feel like the partners come back to themselves for a long time."

> I paced back and forth as I was waiting to go to the OR. Our midwife was my rock, stabilizer, and rational mind to rely on. All I kept thinking was, oh shit. Oh shit. OH SHIT.
> —COBALT, PARTNER OF ALISSA (2011/HBC, WESTERN U.S.)

> I was in such denial that my brain couldn't convince me that a cesarean was actually going to happen. Our midwife was great in terms of telling me what to expect and providing moral support as my wife was prepped for surgery. I was having a tough time emotionally.
> —JIM, PARTNER OF REBECCA (2012/HBC, SOUTHERN U.S.)

> Even though we scheduled the surgery and I knew what to expect, I was still intensely scared when they wheeled her off and I was left alone.
> —MARY, PARTNER OF JESSICA (2003/HBC, NORTHEASTERN U.S.)

They whisked her away and I was handed scrubs. I needed to be alone and not talk to anyone, so I locked myself in the bathroom. I was angry, sad, and needed to have a good cry, but I couldn't right then. I stayed in the bathroom because I was afraid of what I would say to the midwives and I just needed to get myself in control.
—CHRIS, PARTNER OF BRYANNA (2010/HBC, 2012/HBAC; WESTERN U.S.)

When I wasn't by her side, I just about lost it. Had I done enough to help her, to encourage her, to tell her that I believed in her more than anything else in my life?
—DAVID, PARTNER OF MICHELE (2011/HBC, WESTERN U.S.)

The birth team can try to engage the partner by offering gentle reassurance: "I know you're probably scared about what will happen during surgery. Doctors perform cesareans all the time, so this is a routine procedure for them, but it's not for you. You can still advocate for skin-to-skin contact and delaying your baby's first bath."

Retired midwife Pamela Hines says, "I would talk to the partner about what is happening right now to the mother and what to expect in the OR. I would remind the partner that it's okay to talk to and touch the baby, even while doctors and nurses are working on the baby. I would review their wishes and tell the partner that it's appropriate at any time to ask, 'When can I hold my baby?' and to ask this repeatedly."

If the partner, because of fatigue, negative feelings, or her own emotional state, is not in a space to interact with the birth team, she can use this time for personal grounding practices such as stillness, prayer, or breath work. A partner can also make a quick phone call to an understanding and supportive friend, take a shower, brush her teeth, or get the camera ready.

Masked and anonymous
Depending on the level of urgency in the OR, there can be seven or more hospital personnel, plus residents, who are all masked, anonymous, and focused on their tasks. In this situation, it's nearly impossible for a mother to make a human connection. Consider Carol's story at the start of this chapter and the extreme and sudden loss of the attentive care she had received from her midwives during her home labor. Due to the chaotic sit-

uation, her normal abilities to find comfort, connection, and safety were gone, and she was plunged into the stress response. This amplified the atmosphere of an alien environment, attended by faceless providers who lacked resonance with her.

Mothers we interviewed shared different ways they tried to make a connection with the people who were about to first touch their babies. Some said they played music in the OR as a way to unite them with hospital personnel, or they asked for a moment of silence before surgery began. Some non-medicated mothers walked to the operating room so the hospital staff had the opportunity to see them as a people, not as patients on a gurney.

> When I got to the OR, I said to every single person, "This is my baby. I want you to say hi to my baby, please touch my belly. He is present and he can hear you." I am grateful I did that.
> —RACHEL (2009/HBC, WESTERN U.S.)

In addition to experiencing disconnection with masked strangers in the OR, mothers recounted doctors making insensitive comments during the cesarean about their ability to vaginally birth. In the operating room, a mother is wide open and vulnerable because of both the physical process of labor and the act of surgery that renders her immobilized and powerless. Women's health physical therapist Tami Lynn Kent describes the energetic doorway that opens in a woman's body during birth, making her even more penetrable by hurtful comments in the OR: "The negative comments and imprints go in deeply. Everything people say, subtle body language, if providers are worried, if there's fear in the room—all those things get imprinted strongly for a woman." Sensitivity to the fact that, as a homebirth woman, she has had to adjust to a sudden change of plans, and may be feeling vulnerable and shameful, goes a long way towards the mother experiencing less trauma.

> During surgery, the doctor told me there was no way a baby would come out of my pelvis. I know this woman was making shit up, but I've got to tell you, those words, said during a time of trauma, were so powerful. Some of the emotional healing I've been doing over the past two and a half years has been working on my belief that I'm fundamentally flawed. I mean, that's the assumption you're probably going to have anyway after an HBC, but I had a

doctor tell me that I'm basically not good enough to give birth. That's been
really hard for me.
—BETH (2009/HBC, WESTERN U.S.)

Alongside the disappointing interactions with hospital personnel, many women reported an almost equal number of angels: doctors, midwives, and nurses who went the extra mile for homebirth cesareans, sometimes at the risk of losing their jobs, to accommodate the wishes of mothers. HBC mother Jaime shares this note that her husband wrote to the hospital about a specific nurse who offered excellent continuity of care: *Thanks to her help and support, we were able to understand more clearly each step of the process. She went above and beyond the call of duty and became a consistent source of comfort during our time at the hospital. It was clear that she was our advocate and guide through a procedure we had not expected.*

My anesthesiologist was like a doula in the operating room. All I wanted was a waterbirth in my living room, but there I was having my baby in an operating room. He helped so much by giving me a shoulder rub to help me relax, feeding me ice chips when he wasn't supposed to, and compassionately holding my arms as I shook.
—BRANDY (2011/HBC, MIDWESTERN U.S.)

I clicked into postpartum psychosis. I told the nurse that I hadn't seen my baby yet and I didn't know if she was alive. My husband was gone, I was alone, and the nurse said, " I could lose my job for this, but I'm wheeling you into the NICU."
—ELLIE (2006/HBC, 2010/HBAC; WESTERN U.S.)

Voices from the operating room

In pregnancy I had a dream about lots of blood and a masked person who held up a baby with black hair. In the OR, I watched this dream unfold. I wondered if I knew this would happen all along, or if I had created this situation. I still struggle with those two ideas and I'll never know the truth.
—KIM (2001/HBC, MIDWESTERN U.S.)

During my first HBC, I started panicking when my husband brought my daughter to me. I couldn't understand I had a baby because I was losing my mind. I

couldn't breathe and was threatening to kill someone. It was complete insanity. In the end they knocked me out because I was hysterical. I don't remember waking up in the recovery room. I don't remember the first time I held her. I don't remember seeing her face, holding her, touching her.
—KORIN (2006, 2012/HBC; WESTERN U.S.)

For a few seconds, the entire world stopped, and the three of us were the only humans on earth. This was the most horrific birth I could have imagined, yet this was the most magical moment of my whole life. But like most wondrous moments, they are just that: moments. Quickly, I became hyperaware of the surgery taking place again.
—ALEXIS (2011/HBC, MIDWESTERN U.S.)

He didn't smell like anything and I realized it was because they cleaned him. During pregnancy I had nightmares that I had to give birth in a hospital. In the dreams they took the baby away and the nurse guided me to a room full of newborns and told me to find him. I was on an endless search for my baby, and I knew that if I could just smell the birth on him, I would know who he was.
—ANN (2011/HBC, MIDWESTERN U.S.)

I pictured this great homebirth where I'm lying in my bed, snuggled up and nursing all cozy and warm. Instead I'm on a cold table, violently shaking and wide open. My bladder was cut during the surgery and I lay on the table for three hours waiting for the urologist to fix it. My baby and husband stayed with me but I didn't get to hold her because I was shaking.
—ASHLEY (2011/HBC, SOUTHERN U.S.)

In the video of me in the OR I'm smiling, but I was actually very scared and nervous. I didn't know what to expect and I was so sad that this was how it was going to happen. I felt alone for a lot of it. I wasn't asked how I was doing until after we got out of the operating room.
—CHRISTINE (2012/HBC, WESTERN U.S.)

We had originally agreed that if we had to do a c-section, Gary would go with the baby and do skin-to-skin. But because I could feel every stitch as they started sewing me up, I needed him to be there for me, so she was taken away. I still feel guilty about the time she was away from both of her parents so early in her life.

While not the moment I had anticipated, we did have our first moment as a family. Gary told me all about her as I looked at her. He brought my attention to her full head of hair and to her big, alert blue eyes darting around the room. I'm glad that he did, as I was too disoriented to focus on any of those things myself. Without him talking me through the experience so patiently, I would have completely missed seeing my newborn baby in front of me.
—LEAH (2012/HBC, WESTERN U.S.)

Voices from partners

The birth was bittersweet—I was excited to meet the baby but at the same time it was foreign and weird. I couldn't take my eyes off the surgery.
—CHRIS, PARTNER OF BRYANNA (2010/HBC, 2012/HBAC; WESTERN U.S.)

It was an odd mixture of feelings. I saw my baby on the warming table and I was overjoyed, but then I saw my wife on the operating table with her eyes taped shut, tubes down her mouth, and doctors doing things to her body. It was an unusual feeling to feel joy and sorrow at the same time. I was terrified as I waited for her to wake from general anesthesia. All the horrible things went through my mind as I waited—what if she never wakes up or my baby dies.
—JAKE, PARTNER OF CAROL (2012/HBC, WESTERN U.S.)

The OR was a horrible experience for me. Alissa had her arms spread wide in a Jesus on the cross position, we were behind a screen and couldn't see a thing. We heard doctors talking and tugging on her body. They were so disconnected from the person they were cutting open. I just focused on Alissa, touching her, talking to her, being with her. I was feeling grounded, fierce, protective, and completely exhausted.
—COBALT, PARTNER OF ALISSA (2012/HBC, WESTERN U.S.)

For the last month of her pregnancy we knew she needed a cesarean, yet nothing could have prepared me for seeing her so helpless and sad. I expected that I would be better able to take care of her, but the reality was that I couldn't. The experience was just so overwhelming.
—JASMINE, PARTNER OF CHRISTINA (2008/HBC, NORTHEASTERN U.S.)

Cesarean is an initiation

Homebirth women find satisfaction in the active roles they plan for their births, and believe that an out-of-hospital birth will be the ultimate route for carrying them across the threshold from maiden to mother. When pregnancies end with cesareans, these same women sometimes view their births as a kind of death rather than a triumphant entrance into motherhood.

When you consider the initiation phenomena, it's conceivable that an initiation actually does require a death in identity and beliefs. Birthing from Within founder Pam England suggests:

> She's going to have pushed her body as far as she can, and maybe even further than she should, to try to create an experience she internalized as ideal. In doing so, she has most likely put herself up to her own last threshold. That is what initiation is all about. It happens when there is a death, whether it be psychic, spiritual, or emotional—the death of an old self, the birth of a new self.

> By doing all the work of labor, even if it didn't culminate in the outcome she wanted, that giving of herself, giving everything she had and then some, going past her fears, past her doubt, past her physical endurance—that is her initiation by scalpel. An HBC mother has paid the price for her initiation with the death of her homebirth dream.

> *I expected birth to be a rite of passage from the easy, responsibility-free life of the childless to that of the strong and determined mother. Instead, birth didn't just try my resolve—it destroyed it. It obliterated me. It was a birth, a death, a re-birth, and an initiation all in one.*
> —Kate (2012/HBC, Southern U.S.)

When homebirth mothers are able to recognize their cesareans as a true initiation, and can distinguish their moments of power from their moments of collapse, they can begin to see that a passage into motherhood by scalpel is a potent way to cross the birth threshold.

It took months for me to recognize my own power and my place as Mother. The Rumi quote that circles around cesarean pages, "The wound is where the light enters" was my first clue, even before I reconnected with my faith. I could not learn what I needed to learn with my eyes or ears or hands. It simply wasn't getting through, so it found its own way in.
—KATE (HBC/2012, SOUTHERN U.S.)

The golden hour

The idealized entrance into motherhood also includes the magical first hour after birth. Women preparing for out-of-hospital births are inundated by websites and natural birthing books with images of blissful mothers gently nursing their vernix-covered newborns and appearing to bond instantly. Along with these pictures are research studies citing the importance of the first hour after birth as imperative to successful bonding.

The mother's anticipation of the early moments can set her up for disappointment after an HBC because, in most hospitals, cesarean mothers have to wait minutes and sometimes hours for their first contact with their babies. Even if they are able to hold their babies immediately after surgery, they may be too exhausted or confused to remember or be fully present for them.

I thought, well, that's it, we're completely fucked now, our shot at bonding is irretrievably lost. No matter what happens, we will never achieve the same closeness that "normal" mother-child pairs would. I figured my son would believe the world was a cold, cruel place and have trouble trusting others. I felt like it was a miracle that we were able to breastfeed at all. I was sure all was going to be lost because we missed out on the immediate postpartum time together.
—ANN (2011/HBC, MIDWESTERN U.S.)

There I was, on the operating table, looking at the clock and watching my golden hour pass me by. I started to resent that everyone else got to hold and touch my son before me.
—LUISA (2011/HBC, WESTERN U.S.)

He was skin-to-skin with me and he nursed right away. Though I had to wait an hour, I still had my first moment with my baby.
—BRANDY (2011/HBC, WESTERN U.S.)

HBC mother Sara shares these encouraging words for all mothers who "lost" their golden hour:

> Nothing was imprinted on him before you, Mama. I promise. He was a tiny egg cell inside of you first and foremost. Your voice was the first one he heard, and the most consistent one he listened to each and every day *in utero*. He felt your touch every time your hand rested upon your belly. He stewed in, drank, and breathed the amniotic fluid seasoned with your scent and biological makeup. Other hands may have first touched him on the outside and new voices assaulted his senses, but all the while he was searching for you—his one and only birth mother.

Once mother and baby are alone, away from interference, they can recreate that missed time by snuggling in bed skin-to-skin. Smelling, touching, tasting, hearing, and seeing each other helps initiate bonding. For mothers who are unable to feel instantly connected with their baby, it may take time, sometimes months or even years, but a connection will form between the HBC mother and child.

> *People don't talk about not instantly bonding. It's an expectation that you will feel an amazing motherly bond the moment you lay eyes on your baby. But I didn't feel anything after birth. I was so busy trying to make sure nothing else went wrong, that I didn't pay attention to what was right. Once I realized I wasn't bonding, I tried everything—birth reenactment at home, skin-to-skin, licking him so I could taste, smell, and absorb his essence. Nothing worked. I spent two years suppressing joy because I didn't feel I deserved it and that prevented me from bonding with my son.*
> —LIBBY (2011/HBC, 2013/VBAC TRANSPORT; MIDWESTERN U.S.)

Meredith Small, professor of Anthropology at Cornell University and author of *Our Babies, Ourselves; How Biology and Culture Shape the Way We Parent,* diffuses the myth that bonding mainly occurs in the first hour after birth: "Our notions of bonding have been influenced, wrongly, by research with geese. Humans are not geese; we are primates with complex social lives. Our bonding comes from time together, looking, touching, smelling, talking, and getting to know our babies as they get to know us. It happens from long-term daily and nightly connections."

A mother will never know how she will feel about her birth—some women fall in love the instant a line appears on the pregnancy test, others when they feel the first kick, and still others well after birth. Every mother reacts differently to birth, and it's important that midwives, doulas, and childbirth educators prepare women for a wide range of emotional reactions—from tears of joy at the first glimpse of baby to disconnected exhaustion. Women should know to expect the full gamut and that anywhere in between is normal and acceptable, and eventually will feel manageable.

Immediately after surgery

HBC mothers live in two worlds, straddling the identities of wounded warriors and nurturers. They're confused among the chaos of the post-surgery care and trying to mother a newborn. Their journey is forgotten by others soon after surgery—the emphasis is now on the newborn. Mothers receive medical attention after a cesarean birth but rarely emotional triage.

> *There was a disconnect about the surgery, as if it had not happened, and we didn't speak of it at all. No one asked me what it was like or how I was doing. All the focus was on the baby. My birth team attempted to distract me by diverting my attention to my beautiful daughter and my advent into motherhood.*
> —RACHEL (2013/HBC, WESTERN U.S.)

Continuing emotional care immediately after surgery, the birth team can stay physically connected to the mother, offer gentle compliments on the amazing job she did and the choices she made. Before taking their leave, they can remind the mother that they are still her care providers and that she can call them at any time for support. Telling the mother that they will be back within 24 hours and writing down their schedule of hospital visits is important since she often won't recall specific details after surgery.

Before the partner begins making phone calls announcing the birth, or falls asleep because of exhaustion, the midwife or doula can ask for a few minutes of his attention. The birth team can refer to the family's Plan C and ask if the names listed are still the best ones for him to call to bring items they left at home or deliver a special meal. It's here, immediately after surgery, that the postpartum support network can be activated if the family is ready to receive that help. Ensuring other details are taken care of sets the stage for the next steps in a mother's journey and the partner's ability to support her.

Birth Professionals' Quick Guide to HBC Birth

- Use the four points of centering—connect, touch, ask, narrate—throughout the cesarean decision and birth.

- Advocate for the family to have alone time before making a conscious cesarean decision.

- When non-emergent, use desires from Plan C as a negotiating tool before consenting to a surgical birth.

- While the mother is prepped for surgery, support the partner through gentle guidance.

- Remind the mother that bonding happens over time, not just during the first hour after birth.

- Continue to focus and care for the mother in the recovery room or when hospital policy allows for first visitors. Leave written instructions and reminders for the family.

- Help the partner activate the family's support network from Plan C.

Low Flap Transverse Incision, Just Past Midnight

for the doctor who is known and praised for his minimal,
aesthetically pleasing scars

Not even my husband has seen the inside of my uterus,
not even I,
and you
held it handled it cut it opened it squeezed it took from it, twice.
And I want to know:
Did you breathe like you were in a temple
and did you see the light that overflowed the room
and did you hear the song humming inside
as you stopped the blood
and did you see the goddess step down the mountain
to make sure you were doing your job right,
her long hair like tree roots
so thick you would hurt your fingers trying to get in,
and did you know you were touching holy
and did you think about getting home to bed
and did you hold my baby like he was God you were holding
and did you imagine how you came from a cave just like this
and did you feel your hands going into your own mother's body
and did your pulse feel my pulse
and did you take a deep dark breath
with what you saw?
Do you know what you took?
Later that morning when at last your hand slipped beneath your own soft pillow
did your fingertips remember what they felt inside me
and could they say
with any kindness,
or certainty,
where that thing now was
and whether I would ever get it back?

—Written by Claudia (2009/HBC, Western U.S.)

Chapter 6

This is my experience, and it's gonna be fine

We had the most ideal pregnancy, and I thought the birth would be ideal too. It was around 42 weeks when I had a scary dream and woke up feeling like it was time to go to the hospital. My midwife met us there, which was a relief because I didn't have a relationship with the doctors or the hospital. Being there was intimidating, and I felt like the nurses were already judging me. That really set me off and made me feel extremely inferior. I just remember thinking that I did not want my baby born in a room with strangers.

The baby's heart rate dropped during a contraction and everyone went into panic mode. The nurses rolled me over onto my hands and knees, then on my side, and I was handled like a cow. They decided I needed a cesarean and they rushed me to the operating room. Then the doctor settled everyone down, saying the baby seemed okay now, and he wheeled us back to the labor room. During the next contraction, the baby's heart rate dropped, and the doctor said we actually did need a cesarean, so we went back into the OR.

I had a few moments with Christian before I went into surgery. We were really upset and crying, but then I thought, "This is what's happening, this is my experience, and its gonna be fine." In the surgery, the anesthesiologist was really cold, the doctors were talking casually, and I felt anxious. I was lying there wondering if the baby was okay, but they didn't say much until she was born. I was so frustrated because I wanted to hold her right away, but instead they were taking her footprints.

I don't feel traumatized by what we went through. I was pretty sad and disappointed about it, but I realized sometimes it's just what happens. I'm the kind of person who rolls with things, and I just like to experience life. Plus, my midwife had said prenatally there would be things about my birth I would have to grieve—the birth may not go the way I want, my baby might not look the way I want. That was really good for me to hear.

—ANNIE (2009/HBC, 2013/VBAC; WESTERN U.S.)

Many women are devastated by their homebirth cesareans and struggle to gain footing as new mothers, while others seem to integrate the experience with feelings of sadness, regret, or disappointment but not trauma. There is tremendous value in examining some of the complex factors that mitigate women's grief, and building on those valuable nuggets of knowledge to help all HBC women understand and find value in the births they experience.

No dividing line

Following an HBC, mothers might wonder if the emotions they are experiencing as a result of their births are normal, whether they feel calm, devastation, or anger. Wendy Davis, PhD, psychotherapist, and the executive director of Postpartum Support International, suggests, "There is no dividing line between women who will and won't experience birth trauma. Women who have experienced trauma are always looking for that delineation, they are finding a way to judge and compare themselves, and they will discover that not only did they have this harrowing HBC, but others who have aren't even traumatized."

While certain risk factors can point to a woman's higher chance of birth trauma from an HBC, there exists no algorithm for determining where on the spectrum HBC mothers will fall between being deeply traumatized by their births and feeling sad but accepting of the outcome. When interviewing mothers, midwives, and mental health professionals, we discovered some common factors among HBC women who report being non-traumatized by their births. These elements are broken down into two broad categories, the internal terrain of the mother, and her external terrain.

The internal terrain

The ways a woman deals with an unexpected and stressful change of plans, such as an HBC, depend greatly on her internal terrain. This internal landscape involves her innate temperament, her base of knowledge, and her expectations about childbirth, plus her emotional, spiritual, and psychological coping mechanisms. Some of these factors are under the conscious control of the woman, such as the amount of information she seeks about birth and cesareans. However, some of these factors are inherent personality traits, which are not easily adapted or manipulated.

A few women we interviewed described themselves as naturally easy-going, which seemed to make their HBCs less traumatic. This "go with the flow" attitude is known as *cognitive flexibility*, and it allows for easier mental adaptation to unplanned and even undesired events. A laboring woman with greater cognitive flexibility might find that when her birth team suggests that she transport to the hospital, she may initially be upset or angry but then over time, she may become more accepting of the new plan. Arriving at the hospital, she might labor for hours, building high hopes about pushing her baby out and into her arms. When the OB/GYN later recommends a cesarean, she once again feels great disappointment, but when she has some time to process this new information, she is able to move ahead with this change in plans feeling that everything will turn out for the best.

> I tend to be naturally upbeat. It's hard for me to dwell on my sadness.
> —Julia (2011/HBC, Western U.S.)

> As I go into these big life events, I try to keep myself open to not being attached to exactly how things will unfold. There are infinite possibilities and I'm not going to attach myself to specific details. For my birth, I just wanted to make the healthiest choices for our baby. Perhaps because of this, I had less to grieve when my birth didn't turn out the ideal way.
> —Rachel (2011/HBC, Western U.S.)

> I find that the women who can move on from an HBC went into it with openness. I notice those women are better able to find themselves, move forward, and not be lost in what didn't happen.
> —Corrine Porterfield, Maya abdominal therapy practitioner, Western U.S.

Some women look ahead to birth as not only an opportunity to cross the threshold from maiden to mother, but they also look forward to experiencing the raw and unpredictable power of their bodies. Modern life presents few chances to discover our innate potential and limitations, and birth affords women that rare peek. When women have an understanding of their lack of control and can yield to their birth's own roadmap, they may have a deeper perspective for processing an HBC, which can also serve as a solid platform for beginning life as a parent.

Acceptance means saying "I don't know what will happen." After transport, we tend to think about epidural, cesarean, and that it's all downhill from there. But the process of acceptance also calls for non-judgment. That means that we don't make assumptions about what happens next, we only know what is happening now. This is what it means to be present.
—TINA LILLY, PSYCHOTHERAPIST, WESTERN U.S.

Cesarean happens

A few women we interviewed approached their births with an acceptance that hospitals and cesareans are sometimes needed for women to safely birth their babies. Whether this knowing came from working in the medical profession, a childbirth preparation class, or an innate understanding of how birth works, it helped these women feel less shame and self-blame when they did need to engage the medical system.

I went into this birth with the understanding that cesarean was a possibility and that it wouldn't be a failure on my part. I fell into the middle ground of appreciating interventions, hospitals, and homebirths for what they each can offer. That helped going into it feeling like whatever happened would be okay.
—ANNE (2010/HBC, WESTERN U.S.)

I always said that I was trying for a homebirth and if it didn't work out, the hospital was only 10 minutes away.
—RACHEL (2011/HBC, WESTERN U.S.)

Having a little faith

Some women draw upon spiritual faith to help work through their feelings of disappointment after a cesarean birth. Sara planned an unassisted homebirth with her first baby and says the first few weeks after she brought him home from the hospital were emotionally difficult, and she experienced grief about the birth. But then, while watching a televised sermon, she had an epiphany. Sara recalls, "I realized its okay for me to enjoy my baby. Its okay to let go, he's going to be fine. It's going to be all right, we will get through this. That was an important moment for me."

This spiritual foundation can help women access their faith, providing reassurance and opening the door for discovering meaning in a homebirth cesarean. Corrine Porterfield, a Maya abdominal therapist, says, "There is a deep trust within each of us. If we could tap into this and be open to it and trust that there is a divine wisdom, it would be easier to move on after something difficult." For some women, like Sara, this message of hope and inspiration is what enables the emotional healing to begin after a difficult birth.

The external terrain

External factors, or those things that were outside women's mental and emotional control, sometimes influenced the non-traumatic experience of their births. The most commonly reported element was the care women received from their midwives, partner, doula, or the hospital staff. Specifically, women appreciated respectful treatment at home and in the hospital, maintaining a solid connection with their partner and birth team, and having clarity on the decisions being made. When these aspects of a non-traumatic HBC carry over from home to the hospital, women are more likely to have a smoother transition through their cesarean birth.

Wendy Davis summarizes the optimal situation for an HBC mother: "Women say that they knew cesarean could happen so they talked to their midwives about it ahead of time. And they say that usually one person, the doula or midwife, stayed with them throughout the birth." When women are prepared for the possibility of a cesarean and are offered tools to plan accordingly, and they also have the attentive care of their birth team, there is less likelihood that they will be devastated by an HBC.

Treated with respect

Women transporting to the hospital sometimes anticipate poor treatment by hospital staff who may judge them for their out-of-hospital birth choices. When the hospital staff acknowledge the emotional challenges a woman is facing, validate her fears, and treat her with dignity, then the mother's hospital experience can be less devastating. Additionally, women reported that when they had a chance to talk to their OB/GYN and make shared decisions, they felt like the process was more collaborative, resulting in a less difficult birth experience.

> *Everyone at the hospital was very kind, especially the nurses, and that was the most important part of what made my experience non-traumatic. I didn't feel like they had a bad attitude about me because I was a homebirth transfer. It wasn't an emergency situation, so we had time to consult with the OB, prepare*

emotionally, and work together. It was bright, sterile, and completely different from being at home, but overall I feel like it was a good experience. I have sadness and lingering questions, but I don't feel deeply traumatized.
—ANNE (2010/HBC, WESTERN U.S.)

If the hospital staff hadn't been so welcoming, supportive, and non-judgmental about choosing a homebirth, it could not have been the same sacred experience.
—KORIN (2006, 2012/HBC; WESTERN U.S.)

Staying connected to the birth team and partner

Pregnant women planning an out-of-hospital birth spend months building a trusting relationship with their birth team, and they benefit when that bond continues, particularly when a change in birthing plans occurs. Some women cited not feeling traumatized by their HBC because they were able to maintain a strong emotional connection to their midwives or partner throughout the labor and cesarean birth.

My midwife provided me with excellent support the whole time and she is the reason my c-section went as well as it did. My husband and I are private, and she was good about recognizing that.
—JULIA (2011/HBC, WESTERN U.S.)

My emotional recovery was fine because I didn't feel like my care was mismanaged, even though it was an emergency.
—SARA (1997/HB, 2006/HBC, 2008/VBAC; WESTERN U.S.)

For HBC mother Maia, the care she received from her birth team made all the difference in her ability to come to terms with her birth. Returning home three days after her cesarean, she was exhausted and distraught. She says, "My midwives visited daily and really took care of me. I knew I could contact them whenever I needed, and I did call them many times during those early weeks. I think that made it a non-traumatic experience."

The support and attentiveness of the partner is another critical component for fostering a better HBC. In the event of a homebirth cesarean, women desperately need their partner's unwavering stability and reassurance, and when that is present, they can safely surrender to the birth experience. Afterwards, women need partners to listen and allow them to process the birth without placating, interrupting, or dismissing any emotions. When the mother feels this support from her partner and her birth team combined, she will be surrounded by compassionate care that allows her space to explore and process her feelings.

> My husband was very supportive throughout the whole birth. He didn't try to influence my decision, but he was right there helping me process the questions. After the birth, I needed to talk about it a lot and he was a good listener.
> —ANNE (2010/HBC, WESTERN U.S.)

Healthy mom, healthy baby is the priority

A few mothers we interviewed said that they were satisfied to come through their HBC with good health for themselves and their baby. Many HBC mothers bristle at the "healthy mom, healthy baby" comment but some women find that, in the end, they were ultimately able to accept the loss of their homebirth experience in lieu of good health for themselves and their babies. These women view the birth process as less of a focal point than the outcome, and that can help them to put their unwanted HBC into perspective.

> For me, a healthy baby and a healthy mom is the most important thing.
> —PATINA (2013/HBC, MIDWESTERN U.S.)

> I had a healthy baby and I was fine. There wasn't a lot of emotional recourse for me—I felt solid.
> —SARA (1997/HB, 2006/HBC, 2008/VBAC; WESTERN U.S.)

> A cesarean is not the worst thing that can happen. It doesn't mean that I'm not still sad about it, but, at the same time, having a healthy baby does matter.
> —JULIA (2011/HBC, WESTERN U.S.)

It is clear that women's coping mechanisms, knowledge, expectations, and the support they receive from those around them all play a significant role in allowing them to move through their experiences without trauma. When all these factors are in alignment, sometimes women can find the silver lining in a birth that deviated so far from their original expectations.

From Maiden to Mother: A Hero's Journey

WRITTEN BY: BETH ROUSSEAU

This birth myth describes a journey that takes the heroine from ordinary life before her HBC, to the Underworld of cesarean birth, and through the depths of personal struggle and achievement.

In a time not so long ago, there was a Woman who heard the call to become a Mother. She saw the Child clearly in her mind, and felt the sensation of new life growing inside her. Soon, through the act of giving birth, she would become an embodiment of the Great Mother, who created the Universe. The Woman imagined herself growing round with the Child, until the day that she would push it into the world with the force of creation. This was the ideal that had been handed down to her for generations.

Her belly did grow round, and with each passing day, the Woman prepared her body and mind for the challenge of birth. She studied books that claimed to know the way. She strengthened through exercise and focused her mind through meditation. She gathered tools like a warrior preparing for battle: a pool of warm water to ease her pain, soft music to calm her heart, and reassuring mantras to give her fortitude. She felt certain she had everything she needed to succeed.

The day came when the labor pains were upon her, and she was ready. The Midwife was at her side, saying, "This is it. You have begun." She traveled deep inside herself, to another plane of existence. She felt herself crossing a threshold to begin her quest. Still vaguely aware of the others around her, she was no longer fully with them. The Mother was now in another place—an Otherworld between life and death. She knew this was where she would finally meet and claim the Child.

She rode out pain after pain, contorting her body. Hours passed. Days passed. She went without sleep. She barely touched food, taking small sips of drink between breaths and cries. Writhing, vomiting, she endured every test of her worthiness to mother, all the while keeping her focus on the magical goal of pushing the Child into the world. When she felt as if her body could stretch no further, the Midwife said, "Now is the time. Push."

The Woman felt her body move the Child down the tunnel of birth towards the light. Each push filled the Woman with the bliss of accomplishment. She felt she might burst from the joy of being one with her ideal of true womanhood.

Then suddenly, the Woman's body seemed to cease its work. The Child no longer moved down the tunnel. The long labor had taken its toll on both of them. The Woman's will was endlessly strong, but her body was weakening. The Child's body was weakening as well, the signs of life appearing fainter and fainter. Their bodies were betraying them.

The Midwife came to the Woman's side and pointed towards a new threshold on the path. "This Child is held by forces that are beyond our power," she said. "You must go and see the only one who can free him: the Physician."

She moved in pain as she made her way before the Physician. He looked down at the Woman from his seat of power. For many years, women had come to him to deliver their children. From those who sought his assistance, he demanded submission to his judgment. He told the Woman that a sacrifice would be required of her. He would slice open the Mother's body, rending her womb so he could deliver the Child into the world.

The Woman was stunned. She had trusted the Great Mother to give her all she needed to birth. But the Physician held only to the superiority of his medicine. The Woman must admit that birth was beyond her control, and she must trust in him now. With great love and faith, she bravely laid herself before the Physician.

Her eyes were shielded from the ritual. She dare not move, nor speak, nor breathe. She only waited as her body was torn open by the Physician's blade. She felt the wrenching movements of his hands struggling to free the Child. The smell of burning flesh confirmed the destruction of her body.

Her former self was abolished. Now she belonged to the Child, her Son. She was the Mother.

The Son looked at the Mother with the awe of one discovering the face of love. The Mother spoke, and the Son's eyes grew wide with recognition. He knew her voice as if it had been the voice of the Great Mother herself, for indeed the Mother had been his entire universe. She gazed back at her Son, the one most longed-for and desired. The Mother had succeeded in her quest to claim him.

The Mother's joy was brief as the Son was whisked away. Though the Son was no longer in her sight, she was relieved that the ordeal was over and felt herself succumb to a well-earned rest. But her sleep was haunted by nightmares that something was amiss. She began to wonder why the Son was still away from her. She sought him during moments of wakefulness, only to be told by shadowy figures that the Son was ill and being attended by the Physician. They implored her to rest. But the Mother's strength was returning, and with it came the realization that she and the Son were not yet free. They were trapped by the ones who had promised to save them. The Mother knew her journey would not be complete until she and her Son returned to their rightful home.

The Mother arose to fight the Guardians of the Otherworld, pacing the ground like a caged animal. Her captors told her that she was not yet fit to care for herself and the Son. Every day, she proved her strength to them, passing tests of endurance they placed before her. When the captors were finally convinced, they agreed to let her go, but told her the Son must also prove his strength. Every day he did grow stronger until finally, one blessed day, the Guardians threw open the doors, and the Mother and Son began their journey home.

The pathway back was rocky and confusing. The Mother held her Son close to her heart, focusing on his needs, even as she was injured and bleeding. Every step was agony, but she knew they must keep going. Worst of all, she was unsure how to find her way back. She kept putting one foot in front of the other, dreaming of home. She cried out for help, but knew not if anyone heard her pleas.

A Wise Woman appeared on the path. She showed the Mother how to feed her Son. She listened to the Mother's tale, and comforted her. The Wise Woman pointed the way to home. The Mother was deeply grateful, her hope renewed.

The Mother met other mothers who were also returning home from their own journeys. Some of them greeted the Mother warmly and moved on. Some hurried past without seeing her. Eventually, a few fell into step with her, and they journeyed together. As they walked, they talked about the trials they had encountered and the lessons they had learned. No two women had the same story, but all had been tested. Like the Mother, some had faced the Physician, and knew the sting of his blade. Others had faced the Ring of Fire and felt their children burn out of their bodies. The women saw each other the way that only other mothers can, and they felt stronger together.

In time the Mother found she was once again on familiar ground. She was walking the streets of her village, seeing her friends from her life before her Son was born. People who had never been to the Otherworld would ask to hear the tale of her journey. She told them how she had struggled, and triumphed, and returned with her prize. They began to see her as a guide through the labyrinthine path of the Otherworld. She could not tell these women for sure what they would meet there. But she could tell them that, just as she had been, they would be called to greatness.

The Mother walked in two worlds now: Maiden and Mother, Unknowing and Wise. She would always be both, for her journey had taught her that the path of life is unknown. She held this dichotomy gently in her heart as she and her Son proceeded down the path of their life together.

Chapter 7

The womb room

Coming home was bittersweet. My birth team did a marvelous job putting the house back in order, leaving no traces of my homebirth attempt. But when I walked into my daughter's room where the birth tub had been, I broke down. I dreaded seeing that space and faced it alone, feeling that no one else could understand the emotions I was experiencing.

I didn't want any visitors. I was ill-equipped to care for myself, much less be a host. Having a baby was supposed to be a time of joy and happiness to share with others, but it wasn't for me.

My husband did nearly everything from the time she was born until she was a month old. He handled every feeding using expressed milk from a syringe and took care of every diaper change. I couldn't hold her for long because of the pain on my incision. She bonded to him instantly and, with a non-existent nursing relationship, I didn't feel like much of a mother.

I looked at her and was happy she was here and I loved her because she was my daughter, but I didn't get that unconditional love feeling that people talk about. My job was to birth, feed, and comfort her, and I couldn't do any of that.
—Ashley (2011/HBC, Southern U.S.)

The first weeks after a homebirth cesarean are heavy with the overwhelming challenges of recovering from surgery while caring for a newborn, self-doubt about bonding with the baby, and the isolation felt when partners return to work. Many HBC mothers find that their support network all but evaporates after a few weeks—midwifery appointments taper off, friends and family think the mother's sadness and grief over the birth should be resolved, and the stark reality of staying home with a newborn sets in. Additionally, communication with the birth team may be strained if the mother feels angry, disappointed, or abandoned. This chapter looks at the challenges HBC mothers experience, from the hospital stay until the conclusion of care with their midwives around eight weeks postpartum.

The hospital stay

Midwives and doulas we interviewed reported various HBC support protocols that include visiting the mother in the hospital every day, maintaining
the same appointment schedule as for vaginal birthing mothers, not seeing
the family until they are back home, or calling and texting throughout the
hospital stay but not visiting in person. Mothers additionally reported that
some midwives ended their care with them after the birth, leaving them
rudderless and abandoned.

The care-taking a mother needs from her homebirth team requires visits to
the hospital throughout her stay. If the midwife's protocol is to see a mother
at 24 and 48 hours after a homebirth, then the HBC mother must receive
that same frequency of care. Some HBC mothers may warrant extra hospital visits, like when women are having an emotionally difficult time staying
at the hospital, or are feeling "trapped" by the hospital staff.

> *My midwife stayed through the cesarean, but then she never called or came*
> *back. She ended my care after the surgery.*
> —SAGE (2008/HBC, WESTERN U.S.)

> *My midwife visited me every day I was in the hospital. She even told the hos-*
> *pital tech that came to take my baby's heel prick that it must be done while*
> *I held her. The tech said it couldn't be done that way and my midwife gently,*
> *but firmly, told her to find someone that could do it that way. I would not have*
> *stood up to a hospital worker and would not have known it would be best to*
> *hold my daughter during that process.*
> —JAIME (2011/HBC, MIDWESTERN U.S.)

The way the birth team supports the mother in the hospital is different
from the care she would have received after a home or birth center birth,
but similar tenets remain. If the birth team does not visit the hospital, thus
eliminating continuity of care, the mother may think that it is a reflection
of her "failed" homebirth, and not that the midwife or doula is attending
another birth or otherwise unable to visit. When the midwife or doula is
not able to visit the hospital, it can be reassuring to call and text, provide
the family with an option of a check-in from a backup midwife, apprentice,
or postpartum doula, and to clarify that the mother still deserves care from
her birth team.

Hospital personnel are primarily responsible for the medical care of the mother and child, while the emotional and mental needs of the mother are often lost in the process of ensuring their health is within normal limits. Understanding and appreciating that hospital staff and midwives each offer different skill sets can lead to more comprehensive care for the mother. For example, if a nurse hasn't done so already, the midwife or doula can ask her to teach the mother how to care for her incision. When the mother realizes that nurses can show her how to touch and clean her incision and the midwife or doula can provide emotional support while she begins to explore her abdomen, a mother may more easily welcome each person's unique knowledge base. In this way, nurses can focus on their trained skills—post-surgical assessment—and midwives and doulas can use theirs—in this case, emotional support.

The post-surgery information women receive from hospitals varies greatly, and mothers rely on their birth team to help them fill in the gaps. Some hospitals require mothers to watch a video about cesarean recovery or the hospital provides an informational handout. Many mothers, however, do not receive any helpful information about mobility and caring for themselves. (See Appendix F, Incision Care and Healing after an HBC.)

Midwives and the hospital staff can share the responsibility of informing mothers about the physical side of cesarean recovery. Nurses can teach mothers how to safely get in and out of the hospital bed, and midwives can help mothers translate that information to their bedrooms and rocking chairs at home. Before a mother is discharged, she or her partner can request written instructions from the hospital about pain management, warning signs of infection, and phone numbers to call with follow-up questions, which the birth team can refer to when the mother has concerns.

> I swear I'm not a crazy person, but I was crazy then. At the hospital, the nurses didn't hand me my pain meds; instead they locked the drugs in a drawer, gave me the key, and told me the schedule to take the pills myself. They repeated the schedule a few times, but I didn't understand; my brain was super-fuzzy. I wasn't keeping up with my meds because I didn't know when to take them and no one from my birth team was asking about my pain level or helping me figure out the system. (Note: The hospital Ann birthed at bases its self-administering and self-charting policy on research that supports this

method for better pain control. When asked, a physician with delivery privileges at the hospital explained that their hope is to empower women to take charge of their own pain management.)
—Ann (2011/HBC, Midwestern U.S.)

Midwives and doulas we interviewed said they base their level of communication during a mother's hospital stay on the needs of the client, their own comfort levels around HBC, and their relationship with each family. They were sometimes reluctant to bother new families at the hospital, but they had an eagerness to help when asked. Some midwives felt that by saying, "Call if you need anything," they were giving permission to the family to reach out without disturbing them by being in contact too much. However, for a lot of mothers, an invitation for contact is not enough, as they may need more prompting and permission before they will reach out for help.

> My midwives said I could call, but I dared not. I had already cost them three sleepless nights and couldn't imagine bugging them after I'd messed up my birth. Those feelings came from me, not them. They would've had to contact me to persuade me to ask for what I needed. I didn't have the heart to request even more care when I felt like I sucked so much.
> —Ann (2011/HBC, Midwestern U.S.)

Instead, midwives and doulas can tell a mother that they will call her daily, but she doesn't have to answer unless she wants to. Explicitly saying this shows the willingness on the part of the birth professional to stay connected, and still gives the mother the power to choose whether or not to return calls.

> My midwives visited me every day while I was in the hospital. They told me they were sorry that my birth hadn't gone the way I'd planned and that I worked really hard. They talked a lot about how it wasn't my fault. I was really glad they were there.
> —Libby (2011/HBC, 2013/VBAC transport; Midwestern U.S.)

You're supposed to trust and feel supported by your midwives, not left by them. It took a while for me to understand that my feeling of abandonment was about my midwives never coming back to visit.
—MAUREEN (2009/HBC, 2012/HBAC; WESTERN U.S.)

I had a team of three homebirth midwives that visited me in the hospital. They helped with nursing, answered my questions, and in a very firm but friendly tone of a concerned loved one, insisted to the staff that our baby be given donor breast milk instead of formula.
—CAROL (2012/HBC, WESTERN U.S.)

It would have been nice if they had sent someone over for the 24-hour checkup. They would have done that if I was a homebirther. They dropped the ball in supporting me immediately postpartum. Truly, that was the most traumatic part of my HBC. It felt like this whole group of warm-hearted birthin' buddies had just deserted me for being a failure and screwing up their cesarean statistics.
—BETHANY (2007/HBC, 2011/CS; SOUTHERN U.S.)

Birth announcing

At some point in the hospital stay, mothers begin to tell a birth story to friends and family. They may provide medical details explaining why a cesarean was necessary, focus on the personality of their babies, or share general social media updates. Some mothers feel the need to hide hospital details, while others only speak of their sadness about the birth. No matter what level of birth details they divulge, mothers find the storytelling grueling. Often well-meaning friends and family dismiss the mother's grief or reassure her about the health of her baby, rather than listening to her honest feelings and perceptions of the birth.

I tried to hide hospital details in pictures. I couldn't share the real story until weeks later. Only my family and very close friends knew what actually happened.
—LIBBY (2011/HBC, 2013/VBAC TRANSPORT; MIDWESTERN U.S.)

I posted a picture of us snuggling in the hospital. I didn't add details, but it was obvious we didn't have our homebirth. I was amazed at how gracious my friends were, even the ones who were in favor of high-intervention births were very understanding of how sad I was for having such a drastic change in plans.
—BECKY (2009, 2012/HBC; NORTHEASTERN U.S.)

I let my husband tell people the baby had arrived and that I was sick. I didn't actually have to tell anyone for at least a week.
—SELENA (2003/HOSPITAL BIRTH, 2009/HBC, HBAC/2011; SOUTHERN U.S.)

The birth team can suggest that the family give guidance when announcing the birth: "This morning our sweet, 8-pound daughter was born by cesarean after an unexpectedly long and exhausting labor. We need lots of support while we process this birth experience and will be reaching out to family and friends in the coming weeks." This sets the stage for the increased care the family will require after a cesarean, and might stave off some insensitive comments from friends and family.

At least you have a healthy baby
A prevalent part of the HBC experience is hearing the insensitive comment, "at least you have a healthy baby" from friends and family. The culture of mainstream birth focuses on physical outcomes and, in particular, the avoidance of fetal mortality. Some women we interviewed reported that the healthy baby comments portrayed the hospital birth team as white knights who saved their babies from what might have been a potentially lethal situation, when in fact they saw themselves and their babies as deeply wounded by the hospital.

My body had failed me and I had failed as a woman. Being a birthing doula made it even worse. I hid pictures of us in the hospital because I didn't want to be asked about it. To those I did tell I heard "healthy baby, healthy mama is the most important." It made me angry. No, it wasn't all that mattered. There was so much more.
—MARY (2010/HBC, WESTERN U.S.)

Those comments made me feel unimportant to the point of being disposable. I felt deep anger, and my cynicism rose because so much more mattered to everyone else while my birth had to remain unimportant. My birth, even my own health, didn't count for anything.
—Tracy (2011/HBC, Southern U.S.)

Most HBC mothers understand the inherent gifts of birthing their babies outside hospital walls, and they value their baby's health in a holistic sense, not just that their child made it through the birth alive. These mothers know that health isn't only about a breathing baby; it is a complete sense of wholeness and wellbeing. For many HBC mothers, these comments present a false dichotomy—either the mother loves her baby and is simply grateful he is living, or she has skewed priorities and is focused on the wrong aspect of the experience.

I never felt like he was healthy. All I could think about were the long-term risks associated with cesarean. I felt like everyone was telling me I should be happy because he wasn't missing a limb, as if his mental and emotional health wasn't a factor.
—Libby (2011/HBC, 2013/VBAC transport; Midwestern U.S.)

Of course we're all grateful we have a healthy baby—we make babies because we want to raise them. No one needs to be told they should be grateful for that. That's just stupid.
—Korin (2006, 2012/HBC; Western U.S.)

Healthy baby comments minimize the physical impact abdominal surgery has on a woman's body, her future childbearing choices, and potentially her family size. These comments can result in mothers not seeking help with the emotional pain of their births. Fearing that they will appear ungrateful for focusing on their own feelings, mothers may isolate with their grief while sometimes still needing to defend their out-of-hospital choices.

Instead of acknowledging my discomfort, which is true compassion, people wanted to expel it. Pointing out that the baby was healthy was an attempt to divert attention away from what felt shitty and shine it on something else.
—Ann (2011/HBC, Midwestern U.S.)

Maybe part of the problem with "a healthy baby is all that matters" is that our children deserve more than to just be healthy. They deserve love, appreciation, and celebration. And when we are mourning our homebirths, we are mourning the loss of a happy event.
—BETH (2009/HBC, WESTERN U.S.)

Most of the time, commenters don't mean to diminish the mother's emotions. Because American culture isn't comfortable with the notion of holding space for painful and sometimes messy emotions, many people don't know what to say after an HBC. Commenters may be simply excited the baby has arrived and are confused by the mother's sadness.

Being with a mother who just experienced an HBC is like sitting shiva (the traditional mourning period in Judaism after a loved one dies). *It is one of the most uncomfortable and compassionate things a person can do. To make a shiva call, you remain silent until spoken to by the bereaved, and sometimes nothing is said at all.*
—JESSICA (2012/HBC, SOUTHERN U.S.)

To limit a mother's exposure to well-meaning but ultimately offensive comments, either she can avoid making birth announcements to people who may not understand the complexity of her situation, or her partner can make those calls. The mother can also prepare a response to the anticipated remarks that will hopefully stop the person from continuing with more unwelcome opinions. One HBC mother would reply, "She's not healthy, because I'm not healthy," while another mother told her family, "My feelings matter in this situation."

The partner in the early days after birth

Along with emotionally supporting mothers as they announce the birth, partners may be unaware of what it means to fully care for a homebirth cesarean mother, and may require guidance from the birth team. A partner needs clear information about what is emotionally and physically happening for the mother, thereby setting the partner up to better accommodate the mother. When the birth team initiates this conversation, they make it clear that they are still available for information and support even though the family is in the hospital.

Since most partners lack first-hand experience on how to provide post-abdominal surgery support, the birth team can supply written and verbal instructions on how to help the mother as she begins to ease her body out of bed, go to the bathroom, and change clothes. (See Appendix B, Caring for the HBC Mother.)

> *The constant comings and goings of people made it difficult to relax. By the third night, I was so exhausted that I couldn't hear my baby crying or Jaime calling my name from three feet away.*
> —ADAM, PARTNER OF JAIME (2011/HBC, MIDWESTERN U.S.)

The partner is also responsible for ensuring that the mother is adequately cared for, and her wishes for their baby are honored. Accomplishing this may be difficult for a partner in a rested, calm state, let alone a sleep-deprived, adrenaline-driven HBC situation. The combination of pain medication and fatigue will affect her ability to make decisions and advocate for herself. To care for their families, partners we interviewed told us they protected the mother's healing space by hanging signs on doors asking medical residents to not enter, or requesting a different nurse who respected their wishes.

Intertwined with caring for the mother is the partner's own self-care, making sure she is emotionally and physically available for her new family. With gentle reminders from the birth team, partners can call trusted people to stay with the mother while the partner showers, eats a healthy meal, or steps outside for fresh air. The new family can also hire a postpartum doula, even in the hospital, to ensure everyone is taken care of and the mother isn't left alone.

> *Caring for myself was the furthest thing from my mind. But I did play my Nintendo for a few minutes to escape the stress.*
> —GARY, PARTNER OF TRISHA (2007/HBC, NORTHEASTERN U.S.)

> *The exhaustion and shock took its toll on me and my reaction was to shut down. I isolated myself and tried to cope with everything that had happened and that needed to happen. But I didn't cope well. Despite incredible exhaustion, I only slept for a few hours.*
> —MICHAEL, PARTNER OF SERENA (2009/HBC, SOUTHERN U.S.)

Neonatal Intensive Care Unit (NICU)

I was angry that my child was kept from me, and I was having a very primal, animal reaction, pacing my room. I didn't know what else to do. This is what really caused my birth trauma.
—BETH (2009/HBC, WESTERN U.S.)

When a woman, particularly an HBC mother, sees her baby in the Neonatal Intensive Care Unit (NICU), she may blame herself and the choices she made. The partner and birth team can help by providing context and letting the nurses and doctors know the mother's emotional state. If the fight-or-flight or freeze stress response was activated, a mother who experienced this level of trauma is highly susceptible to internalizing criticism for her baby being in the NICU. The partner, friends, family, and the birth team can protect the mother by heading off any comments that imply that the mother's birth choices are to blame.

Understanding that a NICU stay is extraordinarily difficult for parents, the family can request that the hospital provide a patient advocate so they feel they have extra support in the hospital. Midwives and doulas can help the family ask for their right to know what criteria the baby needs to meet before discharge is granted. Though doctors can't know how long stabilization will take, they can be clear about how they are measuring the baby's recuperation process.

Both of our sons were in the NICU for different reasons. I wasn't mobile so I didn't get to meet them until much later. One of the most important things my partner did was handle communications with family and friends. Having a baby in the NICU was devastating for both of us, but my job was recovering from surgery and working to establish breastfeeding, and her job was to handle people.
—DANA (2004/ADOPTED, 2009, 2013/HBC; SOUTHERN U.S.)

Birthing from Within author, Pam England, recommends that when partners are in the NICU away from the mother, that they assure her upon their return that they hurried back as fast as they could. She suggests that "anything wonderful that happened between the partner and baby has to be downplayed for a little while until mom and baby get connected again."

Partners may be tempted to show NICU baby photos to the mother and share them with family and friends, but this can be devastating for a mother who has not yet held her baby. The partner must ask her if she wants to see pictures, if they can be posted on social media sites, and how she wants updates provided to her.

> I feel such deep grief that the first time I really saw my baby was on a camera. I was sitting in the hospital bed tied to an IV and they wouldn't let me leave the room because of the medications. I didn't see him until 16 hours after he was born. I wanted to get my baby, but I believed I couldn't because they told me I had to stay in bed.

> This beginning was the complete opposite of anything we expected. There was no celebration or even a moment with my husband and I looking with wonder at our baby. Right off the bat we launched into a fight to get him out of the NICU. My midwife was telling me there was nothing wrong with my baby, and that was the message I needed to hear, but it was so gentle and subtle that it was lost to me at the time.
> —RACHEL (2009/HBC, WESTERN U.S.)

Welcome home, Mama

Leaving the hospital may be a time of great relief and nervous anticipation. No matter what the mother is feeling, this is when she will struggle with another flood of emotions and physical pain that comes with increased mobility.

The birth team can prepare the family for what the return home might be like by warning about the hours of discharge routines required by the hospital, and mentioning that mothers usually find it emotionally difficult to be back in their home. This is also the time to find out if they want someone from their birth team to meet them at home on discharge day.

> Before discharge from the hospital, I talk to families about starting over when they arrive home as though their baby was just born—skin-to-skin in bed, exploring each other with no other tasks. I talk about how big feelings may come up once they are in their safer space.
> —SILKE AKERSON, CPM, WESTERN U.S.

Some midwives, like Debbie Wong, prefer not to visit on discharge day out of respect for the family's need for rest and privacy, and she explains this to the family during a hospital visit. "There is so much discharge protocol at the hospital that it's usually late in the afternoon before they arrive home and it's exhausting for everyone."

Contrasting Wong is midwife Katherine Bradshaw, who says that her policy is "to visit the hospital the day a family is discharged, take them home, and tuck them back in bed." Because of the emotional impact of a homecoming, many mothers we interviewed said it would have lessened the blow if someone from the birth team had been at their home to greet them. This welcoming can reassure the mother that she did not fail at birth, and alleviate worries she might have about her birth team being disappointed in her. If a midwife or doula is unable to do this, someone from the family's support network can be there as the new family integrates yet another change in location.

> I was an emotional wreck when I came home. The apprentice cleaned our house after transporting, but the birth supplies were still out. That made me awfully sad to see. There I was, back in the room where I failed to progress, failed at birthing, and failed my birth team. I felt like a bad birther. I was walking around in circles, flapping my arms, and crying. Luckily, the apprentice came by and calmed me down, tucked me into bed, and let me cry and talk before she even checked the baby.
> —MAIA (2012/HBC, WESTERN U.S.)

The mother will be grateful to return to a clean home containing no visual reminders of her lost homebirth. A support person can arrive at the home 20 minutes before the new family returns from the hospital. In that time, she changes the sheets, starts a load of laundry, sets the home to a comfortable temperature, cleans up what was missed after transport, closes the bedroom shades, lights a candle, and sets out fresh water and snacks near the bed.

When she hears the family's car, the support person can open the car door to greet the mother as she struggles to stand. She can take her hand, walk her up the steps, and guide her into her home. She can simply hold space as the mother takes in whatever turbulent emotions are coming at her. When the mother is ready, her support person tucks her and baby into bed, just as would happen after a homebirth, thereby bringing the birth experience back to the home. HBC mother Beth says, "I wish someone would have straightened up the house and left me flowers and a note saying they were proud of me."

Coming home was when the grief hit. I was never supposed to come home, to put my baby in a car seat that early, to fret about climbing the flights of stairs to our apartment. I hated the idea of "bringing baby home."

Our house was sort of cleaned up by the birth team. There was a bag of trash in the corner and three loads of laundry from labor. I couldn't lie in bed because we didn't have a single clean sheet and my husband had to go to the laundromat. I wished someone had thought to prep the place.

I also wished my midwives or doula had been there to welcome us home. I felt alone, vulnerable, and incredibly disoriented. It's like I needed someone to re-orient me to my home. I was desperate for a welcoming and reassurance that my home was where we truly belonged, not a place that we fled due to failure.

—ANN (2011/HBC, MIDWESTERN U.S.)

We were met with the smell of being gone way too long: rotten bananas, old pizza, and a neglected cat box. With that smell came a big dose of reality. We had a house to clean, a baby to take care of, wounds to heal, pets to feed, stairs to climb. I wanted to crawl into a hole and die.

Entering our home came with a flood of emotions—happiness, relief, fear, and the sudden realization that it was just the three of us, back to real life. Our midwife didn't meet us there; we drove ourselves home from the hospital, and we had no visitors.

It was triggering to see the tub, and it intensified the anxiety that I was already feeling. It made me numb, made my ears ring and my mind fog. Gary called the woman that rented it to us and told her everything that happened. She stopped what she was doing and rushed over in her gardening clothes, covered in dirt. She drained and disassembled the tub herself and got it out of the house. She then spent half an hour talking to us and helping us process and normalize the experience. She's a midwife at a hospital, and with her own homebirth experience, she had a sense of what we were going through.

After the tub was gone, we finally relaxed. The three of us went into the nursery, Gary sat in the glider with the baby, I stood over him and we cried

tears of relief and joy. That moment was the real end of labor and birth, and the beginning of life as a family. We needed everything gone so that home would feel like home again.
—LEAH (2012/HBC, WESTERN U.S.)

The womb room

When a mother returns home, midwife Sister MorningStar says she needs a bedroom set up with flowers, candles, silence, and someone she trusts nearby. "Imagine the homebirth mom who just had a surgical birth. Maybe her baby was taken away from her and they were separated. She has sorrow and shock and needs to integrate the birth with her baby once they return home. For HBC moms, they need a longer time before they leave their bedroom sanctuaries, what I call the *Womb Room*." Similar to MorningStar, midwife Mary Jackson says she asks the HBC mother to "stay in bed for 24, 48, or 72 hours to do what was missed after the birth, so that they can still have that time together."

If friends and family are unable to respect the fragile space of the new mother and the quiet space of the womb room, they need to be told not to visit. The responsibility for guarding a mother's space falls to partners, but they may need help understanding her desire for quiet and privacy. The midwife or doula can step in and ask if the mother wants visitors and seek assurance that the mother will be cared for by her support network.

I didn't fully understand that Sue needed to create a fortress. I'm very social, so I invited friends over and that was hard for her. It took a while for her to communicate that she didn't want that to happen.
—RACHAEL, PARTNER OF SUE (2010/HBC, WESTERN U.S.)

My husband had people over all the time. I would disappear in my room and refuse to see anyone. I was a recluse just wanting to be with my baby. I cried all the time and my friends didn't get it. I had to hide a lot of what I was going through.
—CHRISTINE (2012/HBC, WESTERN U.S.)

Sister MorningStar knows that everything a postpartum homebirth mother needs, an HBC mother requires twice as much. "She needs more food, more love, more help, and more compassion." She is best served when these are provided to her by her community of family, friends, and neighbors, not just her birth team. If people who agreed to help prenatally can no longer meet their commitments, the midwife or doula can give referrals for postpartum doulas and assist the family in identifying who can coordinate other needed support. This wide network will help the mother build trust with people she will call on many times in the coming years.

Listening in the womb room

During postpartum appointments and when compassionate visitors are with the mother, she needs to be given the capacity to process her experience. "Mom needs to tell her birth story a thousand times," says MorningStar. "Sometimes the same points come out and then suddenly there are new details that emerge because she's been retelling it. Pretty soon all the bad things start to give way to one good thing." The healing begins there. What is the most supportive way to listen to her story? "Don't make a comment, wait for her to continue. And the only question you ask is: *Then what happened?*"

MorningStar talks of a woman's inner emotional terrain—her places of knowing, fears, desires, hopes, and needs—as what is deeply wounded after an HBC. This internal terrain, and the sacrifice of her body and dreams, is something that often goes unrecognized and unnoticed by her family and friends. Bryanna, an HBC mother, says, "It felt like no one understood what HBC mothers go through to get their children here."

Almost all mothers told us they craved recognition for what they went through to birth their babies, and they needed to hear it repeatedly. They wanted to hear it from their midwives, partner, friends, and family. Brooke Noli, a certified birth doula and counselor, suggests that all visitors can compliment mothers. "It's difficult when it doesn't go the way they planned, and women are so hard on themselves. A compliment is such a simple thing. They might not be able to hear the kind words, but if they can, it's great."

Birth team support in the womb room

Even with the best care from her birth team and support network, mothers can still feel neglected. Most midwives we interviewed felt they offer good care to HBC mothers, yet these same mothers reported that the support they received was not enough. Recognizing the care they are receiving can be difficult for traumatized, emotionally vulnerable, and fatigued HBC mothers. This can leave midwives and doulas feeling frustrated, as if they can never help the mother enough.

> It's so obvious that mom is suffering, yet all my attempts to care for her are not enough. It seems not to matter how many hours I spend processing the birth, or how many referrals I make, or how reassuring I am about her physical healing from surgery, it is not enough. Yet, at the same time, she is looking to me, the professional, for advice. Sometimes I feel having someone new to support her, not a family member or a friend, perhaps a postpartum doula, can offer a fresh perspective.
> —Debbie Wong, CPM, Southern U.S.

The birth team or other support people might observe that the new mother outwardly seems to be holding it together, is quiet and shut down, or else just refuses offered help. Perhaps they know that the mother has never needed to accept help before and it's hard for her to ask for it. Using the four points of centering—connect, touch, ask, narrate—can help a mother allow and accept care into her life. It's also important to note that support looks different for each mother. Some mothers may want their house cleaned and the laundry sorted, while others may simply need a trusted friend to lie in bed and watch a movie with them so that they don't feel so lonesome.

> I felt really alone, even with a lot of support. I had deep sadness and was grieving the loss of my homebirth and the entrance into the world I wanted for my son. I felt like I couldn't be a mom because of my limited mobility. To step into motherhood and feel like you can't do anything is hard.
> —Brandy (2011/HBC, Midwestern U.S.)

> My husband and I chose an unassisted homebirth because we are independent people. I desperately wanted to reclaim that lost autonomy, to be a family, a threesome on our own as we'd intended. Where others would have felt abandoned, I wished for nothing more than to be alone with my baby.
> —Sara (2011/HBC, 2013/CS; Northeastern U.S.)

Mothers who feel deep shame and guilt may be unable to accept care when offered, and believe they must prove they can handle motherhood on their own. Tami Lynn Kent offers this advice to mothers:

> Take the opportunity to have a little more love for yourself. Shame is a sign that there is a sense of unworthiness. Birth will go as birth goes. It's not about how good or worthy you are. You start out worthy. You start out precious. You start out beautiful. Your birth experience does not diminish that. You're deserving of full care and full love to help you heal when you have a hard experience.

When mothers view their future bleakly, in addition to working with a mental health professional, midwives and doulas can offer a calming, grounding exercise that validates their experience. Birth teams can also feel better about the care they are giving when they have a tangible tool to offer HBC women. Kent shares the meditation below to use to help restore the energy between mother and child and bring the mother a beginning sense of peace:

> Picture your child the age they are now and then picture them as a newborn on your chest. Breathe that birth energy down your womb, through your cesarean incision, and up to your chest, making an imprint from womb to heart. Let the energy go to your child at the age they are now, and allow it fill up their energy field. Allowing the birth energy to flow through your scar honors their birth process and brings healing as well.

Birth is one moment in the long time of mothering, but the birth energy connection between mother and child always remains. A more complete description of this meditation is in Kent's book, *Mothering from Your Center*.

Follow-up care

The OB/GYN who performs the cesarean is usually responsible for post-surgical care, yet many women we interviewed did not follow up with a hospital medical provider after discharge. Midwives can encourage mothers to see a physician for at least the two-week visit. If they don't want to see the doctor who performed the surgery, midwives can help mothers identify another OB/GYN they may feel more comfortable seeing. If the mother continues care with her midwives, even if she visits a doctor, that leaves the majority of the physical recovery assessment in the hands of midwives.

While midwives are trained in managing post-vaginal birth care, they are not necessarily trained in post-operative care, as it falls outside their legal scope of practice. Repeatedly we heard from midwives that their training in cesarean recovery is minimal to non-existent. Maura Jansen, a graduate of a leading accredited midwifery school, reports that she did not receive adequate training to care for her HBC clients. This sentiment was shared by many midwives we interviewed.

> I'm the primary care provider for my clients post-cesarean, but my knowledge of cesarean recovery is limited. I had a client whose incision became infected and I was the person who had to make that call and take her back to the hospital. It feels really uncomfortable having that much responsibility without having that much knowledge. All of my questions about cesarean recovery are from a midwifery perspective, and I keep looking to OBs to provide that information, but they don't have it because they aren't midwives.
> —SILKE AKERSON, CPM, WESTERN U.S.

When midwifery and doula education programs and workshops teach about postpartum care for HBC mothers, these professionals will be skilled at assessing post-surgical pain levels, and understanding what are normal and acceptable pain levels.

> I didn't ask my midwife for tips on mobility. I was only her second cesarean, so I thought she didn't know. I didn't even give her the chance.
> —NICOLE (2011/HBC, MIDWESTERN U.S.)

Often, mothers want their midwives to examine their incision, offer reassurance if it is healing normally, and provide options to help it mend safely with minimal scarring. The more knowledge birth professionals have about cesarean recovery, the better able they are to answer mother's questions. (See Appendix F, Incision Care and Healing after an HBC.)

Twice I asked my midwife to look at my incision and she seemed put off and didn't follow up with wound or incision care. The only postpartum instructions I received from her were scribbled on a post-it note. I remember feeling slightly guilty and ashamed for asking her to look at it because of how sad she acted.
—LEAH (2012/HBC, WESTERN U.S.)

Another hurdle in gaining adequate cesarean information is that the incidence of homebirth cesarean is low enough that midwives don't have experience examining incisions; when they do, they may not know what is normal. A midwife who sees only a few cesarean scars each year may not feel confident in her assessment skills, and that discomfort will be evident to the new mother.

I don't feel my midwife knew what she was looking for when she examined my incision, but she knew enough to tell me to skip a round of ibuprofen to determine if I had a fever. That's what led us to return to the hospital.
—ALISSA (2011/HBC, WESTERN U.S.)

Workshops and classes that offer midwives and other birth professionals instruction on the physical and emotional aspects of surgical recovery, common incision problems, and pain management can supplement the standard training. Even in the absence of formal training, midwives and doulas can build skills and comfort by inspecting incisions at each appointment. Doing so will help them learn the normal progression of healing scars, and they may also catch a problem early since they might see that the incision looks worse than it did the last time it was examined. This practice also helps the mother normalize her surgery, and perhaps even feel comfortable beginning to touch and form a relationship with her scar. (Visit www.HomeBirthCesarean.org/workshops/ for workshops offered to birth professionals.)

High-stakes breastfeeding
To offset feelings of disappointment or body inadequacy, HBC mothers who choose to nurse want to excel at breastfeeding as a way to reconnect with their bodies, hold on to a vestige of their homebirth dream, build confidence, and prove their competency as mothers.

I already felt like a failure for not being able to birth my own kid, so our nursing success was huge for me as an emotionally recovering c-section mom. Overcoming my negative thoughts was made easier by knowing I was awesome at feeding him.
—ALEXIS (2011/HBC, MIDWESTERN U.S.)

Having such a happy and productive nursing relationship was healing. To give my daughter what she needed restored my faith in my body, whereas not being able to birth her really stole that away from me.
—SUE (2010/HBC, WESTERN U.S.)

Breastfeeding can be challenging to any mother, but for the HBC woman, nursing issues are an added loss stacked on top of the birth experience. Some HBC mothers may encounter a range of challenges: being unable to make enough milk, the baby having an ineffective latch, or discovering that although they wanted to breastfeed it becomes too emotionally triggering because of abuse history or prior trauma. Dave, husband of Courtney, put it simply when he said, "Can't at least this go right for her?"

Lactation consultant Meg Stalnaker explains why the early days of breast-feeding can be difficult for many HBC mothers and babies: "Because of the surgical birth and the pain medications that accompany it, a cesarean born baby is often sleepy, and the drive to seek the breast can be temporarily diminished. Combine that with the mom recovering from surgery and the whole process of milk coming in may be interrupted."

I was embarrassed and ashamed, and didn't want to feed her in public because I felt judged using a bottle. Those feelings intensified when maternity leave ended and everyone expected me to have a breast pump at work.
—CARRIE (2012/HBC, MIDWESTERN U.S.)

I pumped for two and a half months, combining the small amounts of milk I got with formula. I was sometimes spending an hour at a time on the pump and getting mostly blood. When I stopped pumping, I felt relief alongside crushing guilt.
—LEAH (2012/HBC, WESTERN U.S.)

If healthcare professionals understand the common nursing challenges following an HBC, they can proactively assist mothers in building a healthy nursing relationship immediately after a cesarean. (See Appendix G, Breastfeeding after a Homebirth Cesarean.) Lactation consultants can aid an HBC mother by listening to her story, providing her with options like exclusive pumping or donor milk, and supporting her feeding choices. Lactation consultant Melissa Cole notes that emotional grieving is always a component for HBC mothers. She makes it a priority to validate that experience during her lactation appointments. She also helps the mother discard erroneous information from hospital staff, friends, or other people who are not breastfeeding experts.

Mothering, bonding, and HBC
In addition to helping the mother nourish her baby, midwives and doulas must also support the mother as she learns to bond with her baby. She may be reassured to know that bonding takes time and solidifies as she rests, heals, and gets to know her baby and her new self as a caretaker. One of the problems for an HBC mother is that her incision gets in the way of what she may picture as typical bonding behaviors—feeding, diaper changing, baby-wearing, and curling around baby during sleep. These impediments evaporate as the mother's incision heals, but feelings of disquiet about the bond can remain.

> I wondered if I loved my baby less because of the cesarean. I looked it up online to see if I was missing an essential connection. At first, I didn't feel a whole lot of love. I could have felt the same with a vaginal birth, but it shook me—was it because of how she was born?
> —ANNIE (2009/HBC, 2013/VBAC; WESTERN U.S.)

> I didn't have that bond that everyone tells you about with a new baby. That was painful. If I couldn't give birth to him, maybe he wasn't meant to be here. I thought all kinds of awful, awful things.
> —LIBBY (2011/HBC, 2013/VBAC TRANSPORT; MIDWESTERN U.S.)

> In terms of bonding, whenever I looked at him I had this intense wave of guilt. When he cried, I felt like he was yelling at me and was upset about the way he was born.
> —ANN (2011/HBC, MIDWESTERN U.S.)

Birth professionals can normalize a mother's fear over bonding, reminding her that bonding happens over a lifetime. The birth team can also offer resources, such as the Homebirth Cesarean Facebook group, that allow mothers to connect with each other. (See Appendix C, Resources for HBC Mothers and Families.)

Did I let my birth team down?

Just as a mother might worry about the bond with her child, she may also fret over the bond with her birth team. During our interviews, mothers reported concerns that they had disappointed their midwives and doulas by needing a cesarean. Some expressed sadness that their births might have altered their midwife's cesarean stats, while others thought their birth team was upset because they didn't get to attend a vaginal birth.

> One of my thoughts was that I was going to ruin their stats. What if my HBC made their c-section rate move from 7% to 8%? I was going to screw up their pamphlet and that was a concern for me. This projection of my disappointment was a way to avoid really feeling my failure. There was no real reason to think my midwives would be disappointed. It was all me.
> —Alexis (2011/HBC, Western U.S.)

Midwife Sister MorningStar suggests that this need for women to please others comes from our inability as a modern culture to act in instinctual ways that might go against societal norms. Women are taught to be polite and kind, and that can interfere with their innate needs. A mother may refuse visitors at her home because she needs privacy, but at the same time she may feel intense guilt about denying people access to her new baby.

Another consideration is that if a mother is worried about disappointing others, it may be that she is truly disappointed in herself. That projection may cause nervousness about how others might be judging her. MorningStar explains that "when we are apologetic for who we are, that affects everything. We start to get into the mindset of *I hope I didn't let you down.*"

> I felt like I had let everyone down—my baby, family and friends, my midwives, even the homebirth community.
> —Carol (2012/HBC, Western U.S.)

The partner's postpartum adjustment

As the weeks pass, partners find that their focus shifts from the immediate care of the mother and baby, to returning to work and finding balance among home life, their job, and other commitments. Partners shared with us a common desire to move on from the birth experience and focus on caring for their new family in more tangible ways. Partners spoke of learning to be a new parent while managing sleep deprivation, making lifestyle changes, and handling the new mother's physical and emotional needs.

Sometimes returning to work and figuring out this new life requires a compartmentalization of the birth, the postpartum experience, or other challenges brought on by the HBC. The partner may find that the raw edges of the birth become dulled by the mental demands of focusing on his job, or the sleepless nights and relentless newborn care that are a normal part of new parenthood. In order to arrive at work with the ability to be productive, partners often find that they need to lock away and forget the most difficult parts of the experience. While this can be a helpful coping mechanism at work, it means that upon returning home, the partner needs to once again face a mother who has been caring for the baby and dealing with her own grief. When partners are unable to switch back into emotional caregiving mode for the mother, it can be a difficult transition for the whole family.

> I found some clarity once I allowed myself to do things for my body to help process the anger I was holding—massage, soaking in a hot tub, and working with energy healers. It was too easy to fall into the mindset that everything I did had to be built around saving the day. I completely overlooked my own needs and once I got over the guilt of taking care of myself, I was able to be a better partner and father.
> —DAVE, PARTNER OF COURTNEY (2011/HBC, WESTERN U.S.)

In addition, a surprising number of partners shared that at some point before or during the cesarean they feared the mother was going to die. During the labor, partners were functioning on high adrenaline; which, combined with experiencing a mother in a serious medical situation, caused partners to fear for her life. Afterwards, partners felt tremendous gratitude that the mother survived, and baby was healthy. This thankfulness for a new beginning sometimes carried over into a desire to bury the experience and the mother's feelings about it.

Lara Williams, an OB/GYN, puts these feelings into perspective as a provider who works in high-risk situations: "Worldwide the number one cause of death in childbearing women is still childbirth. I think there is a perception that in America birth is "safe" and that hospitals make things worse. This is a narrow view of a much more complicated situation and does not truly reflect what is happening."

> We never had a moment together to process or breathe. Suddenly we were separated and we didn't even get to say goodbye. I realized that if she died in surgery, I would be a single parent. I kept thinking, "A single father? I don't want to be a single father!"
> —GARY, PARTNER OF TRISHA (2007/HBC, NORTHEASTERN U.S.)

> I was nervous about the surgery. It seemed to take forever and it was so surreal. If we didn't have this option, what might happen? Sue might die, the baby might die, they both might die. The whole concept is terrifying to me.
> —RACHAEL, PARTNER OF SUE (2010/HBC, WESTERN U.S.)

Even in vaginal birth scenarios where nothing unexpected happens, some partners feel unable to determine their place in the family. The mother and baby are a dyad, sometimes causing the partner to feel left out, helpless, and unsure where he fits into the nurturing relationship. In some families, the mother is so desperate to bond that she refuses to be separated from her baby for even a few minutes. That can make it difficult for partners to feel like they have a place as a co-parent, and they may end up withdrawing as a way to protect themselves. For a mother, this creates a sense that her partner is inattentive to her needs, and even a sense of resentment over the fact that the partner has the luxury of free time while she is at home caring for the baby.

As the mother begins to wade through her own complex emotions, her partner may or may not engage in the same level of processing. In some cases, the partner may feel deep sadness in how the birth evolved, or feel like he was powerless to prevent the unwanted chain of events that unfurled. The partner may have been deeply traumatized by seeing the laboring mother or baby treated poorly, or in dire medical circumstances. However partners felt around the time of the birth, it's common for them to suppress their own emotions.

I avoid talking about the birth. It's too much to think about.
—JUSTIN, PARTNER OF TERRA (2011/HBC, NORTHEASTERN U.S.)

He wanted me to be okay, first and foremost. He wasn't necessarily upset that the cesarean happened, but he was upset that I didn't get what I wanted and he knew I was sad about it. He still comes from a place of "everyone's healthy, so that's all that matters," but he takes the feelings that I have about it seriously.
—JULIA (2011/HBC, WESTERN U.S.)

In an ideal postpartum situation, both the new mother and her partner have ample opportunity to discuss their evolving emotions with each other and the birth team. Often, though, the follow-up visits with the birth team take place when the partner has returned to work, and it can be difficult to request additional time off to attend these appointments. If the midwives haven't explained why the partner needs to be at the postpartum visits, the partner may not understand the importance of having time to discuss the birth and his feelings about it. In these cases, midwives don't understand the partner's feelings, and an unsettling lack of closure can persist that prevents resolution.

Midwives and doulas can let partners know throughout the prenatal and postpartum care that they value the input and feelings of the partner, and they can request that he attend appointments whenever possible. If in-person visits cannot happen, the midwife can schedule a phone call to address the partner's needs, thereby fostering an open invitation for continued support.

At first I didn't recognize my own needs, so I didn't get a chance to do all the work necessary around my own processing. The realization came when I would suddenly burst into tears whenever we were with our midwives. They did home visits for six weeks after the birth, and it was so great to process some of what I was feeling in the comfort of our own home.
—CATH, PARTNER OF JO (2012/HBC, WESTERN U.S.)

Feedback to midwives

A hallmark of midwifery care is the trusting relationship between mother and midwife. The mother and her midwife move from frequent visits after a birth to a more routine schedule of postpartum appointments. During this time the mother may experience a range of emotions concerning her midwives—from deep gratitude, to feelings of disappointment or abandonment.

> When I was thanking my midwife for her support, she said that's just how she handles aftercare. She visited every day, then every other day, then every three days for weeks, until she saw my health return. She was the person who told me I was being a wall, that I needed to process the birth. She told me to find an avenue—to do something.
> —ALISSA (2011/HBC, WESTERN U.S.)

> They were awesome about calling and checking in to see how I was doing for well past the six weeks of care I was supposed to receive. One of my midwives even asked if they could have done something differently. It was nice to know that they thought about it.
> —LIBBY (2011/HBC, 2013/VBAC TRANSPORT; MIDWESTERN U.S.)

As the fog from recovery, fatigue, and caring for a newborn begins to lift, the strong emotions left behind by the birth are revealed. The HBC mother has been in survival mode for weeks, and she now may look back and begin to realize that she feels upset about the care she received from her birth team.

> When a homebirther has a cesarean, the surgery itself is rarely the trauma. Usually, there is some kind of disruption in a relationship that is the most disturbing aspect to the mother—someone wasn't there, the midwife backed off, and there is now a painful connection with the natural birthing community.
> —PAM ENGLAND, AUTHOR AND FOUNDER OF BIRTHING FROM WITHIN, WESTERN U.S.

> I asked to do a closing ritual with the midwives. It was sweet, but I feel we just covered up things. We never actually talked about the birth.
> —RACHEL (2009/HBC, WESTERN U.S.)

My midwives pulled back emotionally. I got the impression, though I never talked to them about it, that they were afraid that I was upset, so it made the relationship between us more strained. I don't know if they were concerned that maybe I would blame them, or if they just felt bad and didn't know how to address it.
—JULIA (2011/HBC, WESTERN U.S.)

Countless HBC mothers struggle with the idea of providing constructive feedback to their midwives. Some fear their midwives will not remember their births; others worry about "bothering" them since they are no longer in their care. These concerns are in direct conflict with providing feedback, so it can be hard for women to come to a place where they feel ready to share their feelings. As one mother put it, "Since 2006, I've written lots of letters to her, but I haven't sent one."

Over time, my thoughts have become more complicated. A lot of my negative feelings are misplaced—I'm putting them on her to feel better about the role I played. She's my scapegoat. I feel like sometimes in my head, I exaggerate her role and build up the ways she failed me. But a lot of it is real and valid. She really did fail at doing certain things we agreed to. She did contribute to me feeling lost and abandoned.
—LEAH (2012/HBC, WESTERN U.S.)

I told our midwives to make sure they prenatally have the tough conversation about cesarean with moms. One midwife said she didn't want to do that because she didn't want to scare moms or make them fearful of birth. I said, "You know what's scary? Not having the facts and needing to transport when no one has talked to you about it. You owe it to them to have those uncomfortable conversations." And you know what? They started doing just that.
—ANN (2011/HBC, MIDWESTERN U.S.)

Emails to midwives
Here, we offer a glimpse of the type of feedback five mothers sent their midwives.

This email was handwritten at 12-months postpartum and emailed four months later by a woman who felt like she had to bottle up her emotions in order to function as a mother. She explains her conflicting feelings about the lack of response from her midwife: "I didn't invite or request a reply, and at first I was at peace with not hearing from her, but now I feel disappointed and angry about that. And so my healing story continues."

First, I want to thank you for the attentive prenatal care I received. I felt well cared for, and that you had time for me. You were patient and answered my questions and concerns.

Second, due to the high-quality prenatal care I received, I expected the same attentive care during labor and birth.....I expected a greater willingness for whoever happened to be on call to be present with me during labor. My husband and I had never been through labor and we were relying on the birth professionals with whom we had contracted to guide us through the process.... We were in the hospital for 4 days. We heard not a peep from any of my midwives. It was your job to show up. It was your job to check in with me, not to leave and never come back.

At eight months postpartum, this letter was sent by an HBC mother to one of her midwives.

...Once you did get to the hospital, you didn't seem to be present with me. You changed from the person I knew into someone I didn't recognize. I thought that you were supposed to become my doula, to help me, calm me, guide me, and be an advocate for me. Perhaps I assumed wrong, but none of this happened. I felt HORRIBLE each time you answered the phone to tell your daughter you weren't going to be home since things were taking so long.... I was miserable and no one seemed to get it....I wanted help. I needed help. I felt more like an inconvenience than a client whose plan had strayed. I was in the most helpless state and I felt so alone.

I wanted you to know how I felt and what I perceived. It may not be what really happened, or what you felt happened, but it's what happened to me. It's how I was treated and it hurts. I don't trust people easily and I had put my trust in you and in my darkest hour you sat on the side lines on your phone waiting for it to end....

At six weeks postpartum, this email was sent by an HBC mother to her midwife who also attended three of her other births. After each of her previous births, the mother painted her a picture that was representative of her baby. After her HBC she had no will to paint anything about their journey together. Instead she wrote her a five-page letter of thanks.

…When we found out that we were pregnant this sixth time, we asked if you would walk this journey with us. And you did. Though it didn't turn out the way we wanted, there are still some things for which I am thankful. You went above and beyond with home visits so that I didn't have to drag my exhausted self and 5 children to the clinic. Thank you. Having you draw blood in my backyard, because it was way more for convenient for me than trying to juggle getting to a clinic, is a good memory, even if it has to do with blood work. My children know who you are. And you let them be part of the process even when it was less convenient….

At three months postpartum, this email was sent by an HBC mother to her midwife. Some difficult conversations between the two women followed.

…There was one particularly painful statement that came from you. You told me, "Because you are going to get a c-section, I am going to leave." And then I never saw you again until three weeks later. I only got text messages, often that had to be initiated by me—despite the fact my daughter was in the NICU, and that I was still your client, paid in full for your services….

Facebook is a silly thing in which we present ourselves in our best celebratory light, but you didn't mention my birth. There were plenty of successful births posted, but not mine. Is a hospital birth and moreover a cesarean not to be celebrated? Does it mean I failed, and therefore am not worth mentioning?…

Personally and professionally, I felt abandoned by you, and the only reason I can find for it is because I didn't push her out the baby hole. That I marred your statistics as your first cesarean baby of 2012. That I somehow failed you….

Below is the email sent by author Courtney to her midwives Laurie and Kim seven months postpartum.

...Since Lazadae was six weeks old, I've been wanting to provide feedback.... First, I want to be clear that nothing anyone could have done would have changed the outcome of my birth. Lazadae needed to be born via cesarean and though I don't understand this part yet, I needed to have that experience as well. I believe that with my entire being....

...I know it must be hard to transport a mom with waters broken for 50 plus hours, creeping blood pressure, and then a surprise breech—you both handled it well.

Where I needed more support was when I returned home and in the weeks after. As a homebirth turned cesarean mom, I was left floating in an unknown world with no one claiming me. I wasn't a patient of the hospital, yet the two of you weren't helping me figure out how to navigate my surgery. I had to call a friend and ask her how to sit up from a chair, how to cough without feeling as though my incision were busting apart. It wasn't until a postpartum doula handed me a Cesarean Tip Sheet with helpful information about recovery, support, and surgery basics that I learned anything. Where was that tip sheet from you? Why didn't either of you know the best way to remove the Steri-Strips from my incision one week after the surgery?

There were several times when I asked cesarean questions and you didn't know the answers. One time in particular, when I asked how my incision affected fundal height, because you didn't know the answer, it seemed like a good idea to call the hospital midwives and find out. This was something I've seen other midwives do and I didn't understand why it wasn't being done for me. From my perspective, it seems that there is a lack of education about cesareans in general and postpartum surgery care in particular.....

After leaving the sacred bubble the hospital provided for us, I was thrown into utter confusion and grief. There I was, unable to stand up straight or lie down flat and I hadn't slept but a few hours for almost a week. I was frantic trying to manage all the problems I was being dealt. My first priority was breastfeeding and my milk supply. Second was her hips and her harness. Third was my body and its health and recovery and fourth was our midwifery care. I know that during the first week I cancelled an appointment and pushed away your care. I was so distraught and could barely handle anything else. You both gracefully moved aside to let me get the help I needed and you both remained open and helpful when I asked for it.

But then I didn't hear from either of you between weeks two and four. That's two weeks of no communication from my midwives, my midwives who knew the details of my struggle and could only guess the depths of the potential postpartum depression and shock that was brewing.

At what point do you change your protocols when a mom transports? At what point do you call more frequently? At what point do you have a few extra visits or extend postpartum care?...

I won't be your last cesarean mom, which is why I'm providing you with this feedback. Cesarean is a very valid form of birth. By not understanding as much as possible about the recovery process and changing to meet its unique postpartum needs, you risk invalidating this birth experience for a mom. In my situation, I felt this part of my experience was invalidated.

Please know that I send this message not out of anger or malice, but in the spirit of open communication. I want to share my experience so that you can help the next mom.

Birth Professionals' Quick Guide to the First Eight Weeks

- Provide a written and verbal schedule of hospital and home visits.

- Check in via phone and text daily, then taper off as the mother's physical and mental health stabilizes.

- Ensure the partner has written down important information from the hospital.

- Meet the mother at home after hospital discharge, or help arrange for a close friend or family member to welcome her home. Ensure all birth supplies are out of sight.

- Offer extra visits and encourage the family to hire a postpartum doula.

- Help seek commitment from the partner or other support person that the mother will have the care she needs.

- Listen to the mother's birth story, and guide the partner to do the same.

- Examine the incision at each visit.

- Educate the family about normal cesarean physical and emotional recovery.

- Invite feedback at any time and listen with an open heart.

Staples

The stapled woman sneezing
holds one hand to her mouth, the other

her incision. She doesn't laugh
when the staples are out

for months. A year after the staples
she asks her husband

if he remembers. He says *forget.*
She shows him a picture of the staples—

a fence across a meadow.
From the shower she sees her daughter

see the scar, says *the earth opened*
you lifted out.

—Written by Dave, partner of Courtney (2011/HBC, Western U.S.)

Chapter 8

In service to families

It is my personal goal that each woman and family feels empowered through their birthing process. My work as a midwife is so sustaining when I can make the connection that it's not about me, but instead about the family and their accomplishment.

I learned through the family's pain, the confrontation of sitting face-to-face with new parents and hearing that I should have done more to prepare them for their cesarean births. I feel lucky that I was not raised in a guilt-laying family, so I never got mired down in judgment. But it did mean I had to make some major changes in the way I cared for women. That has been the most valuable teaching I have had—that direct feedback from families.

When a birth turns into a cesarean, I go back to the woman. The first impulse of midwives is that it's scary, like you're going back to the scene of the pain. We have to return to that place of familiarity with birth, with death, with all of that brutal stuff. That's nature, that's life. That's midwifery—letting go of the judgment and the guilt. The more contact I have with families, the more at peace and the more repaired I am.

—INGRID ANDERSSON, CNM, MIDWESTERN U.S.

Midwives learn in their training that not only will they employ their skilled hands and quick-thinking minds in their calling, but also their hearts. They sacrifice predictable daily routines and sleep in lieu of witnessing the evolution of maidens to mothers, individuals to families. Kneeling beside the bed, rubbing a laboring woman's back through the night, the midwife knows that her presence and open heart lend comfort and reassurance to the mother. When that labor is long or complicated, the midwife fully devotes her attention to the new family, while she sometimes struggles to hold together her life outside of the client's microcosm. When her client has a homebirth cesarean, a midwife experiences her own complex web of emotions, from relief, to grief, to disappointment or failure. Depending on how the mother feels about the birth and the care the midwife gave her, she may need to reconcile her client's feelings toward her and that can be painful for both. This chapter examines the midwives' experience of homebirth cesareans, and the many layers of impact these births have on a midwife's emotional, physical, professional, and home life.

Homebirth cesarean through the midwife's eyes

Lena answers the phone in the middle of the night, quietly reassuring the first-time mother and assessing how far along in labor she might be. Returning to bed, she lies awake, making mental notes about alternative plans for her own childcare, meals, and appointments. A few hours later, the phone rings again, this time the call comes from the anxious dad, requesting Lena's presence. She quietly packs her bags, then calls her assistant. Before climbing into her car, she stands still for a moment in her front yard, relishing the opportunity to observe what the nocturnal creatures find commonplace.

Arriving at the mother's home, Lena quickly becomes absorbed by the intensity of the labor. She feels an intimate connection to Amy, who seems strengthened by Lena's smiles of approval.

Morning arrives, and Lena steps outside to answer a call from the babysitter, who needs to get to an appointment and cannot take the baby with her. She phones her mother-in-law, who agrees to pick up the baby and drop her off at a neighbor's house. Back inside the house, Lena sits beside Amy, rubbing her back and intuitively knowing the right amount of pressure to apply. The hours melt away into evening and Lena's phone rings. An overdue client reports having mild contractions. She enthusiastically reassures the mom, while secretly hoping her labor will wait just a bit longer.

The nighttime hours bring frustration for Amy; her labor is long and seems to have slowed down. Lena and her assistant have tried countless tricks to allow the mother to alternately rest and also to help move labor along, but Lena begins to doubt that her own efforts are yielding any benefit to the mother. She wonders if she has overlooked something that might reveal the reason behind the stalled labor. Reviewing the chart as the assistant sleeps, she begins to question if she should offer Amy IV fluids. Lena recalls a recent story from a colleague, whose client had a poor outcome for the baby, and considers if she should initiate a conversation with Amy about going to the hospital. She checks in with the weary partner, who shares concern for the mother's waning stamina. His attentiveness and connection to Amy bolster Lena's waning energy, and she offers to brew them both some coffee.

As the night progresses, discouragement and fatigue overtake the house, and Lena gathers everyone to discuss transporting. She expresses her hope for a vaginal birth at the hospital, but her weary mind registers a look of defeat on Amy's face. By early morning, Amy resigns herself to transport; she is exhausted, emotionally drained, and contractions are irregular and ineffectual. Lena feels an unsettling mixture of dread for the family's upcoming hospital whirlwind experience and relief that the mother has consented to transporting.

Lena initiates plans for transport while the assistant helps the confused dad pack and gather items Amy is requesting from her perch on the toilet. She wonders how she will pull herself together to provide support for the family and regrets not napping earlier in the night. The assistant midwife stays behind to drain the birth tub and will meet them at the hospital.

Lena drives in front of the mom and dad, and she walks with them to labor and delivery, vaguely aware that she has not showered, her clothing is rumpled, and bags hang under her eyes. As Amy settles in, Lena shares the medical chart with the nurse, who seems surprised that pertinent information is provided. The mother's expression is one of exhausted resignation, and Lena is unaware that Amy has entered into the fight-or-flight stress response.

Throughout the long hours ahead, Amy dozes with the help of pain medications, the dad snores, and Lena tries to grasp a few minutes of sleep. She leaves the room to call her husband and phones a fellow midwife to see if she can check on her other laboring client.

As the day progresses, Lena sees that a cesarean birth will be needed since there is still little change in her labor, and her heart aches for the loss of the homebirth dream this family will surely experience. Lena feels helpless as the full weight of the decision to choose surgical birth blankets the room.

In her fatigue, Lena wonders what she did wrong, what she did not do right, or if she failed to detect a mal-positioned baby early in labor. She is concerned that Amy is her third transport this month and dreads the thought of facing another peer review. Lena feels anxiety rising in her chest as she imagines describing yet another cesarean to a group of midwives who might find her inept or inexperienced. She also second-guesses her decision to transport Amy, maybe they could have stayed home.

The baby is born by cesarean an hour later and Lena waits in the labor room after she finds a cup of coffee in the cafeteria and brushes her teeth. The mother and baby return to the room, and Lena is relieved to see them both. She helps the baby begin her first feeding at the breast, while encouraging the dad to stay close and connected with his family. Lena mourns their loss of the intimate first moments they may have had after a birth at home—she knows what might have been for them. Once the new family is settled, Lena hugs the mom and dad, promising to return in the morning.

The midwife-mother bond

> Why aren't there books about the sorrow of a midwife during a cesarean? Because it breaks her heart too. Where are the books about the heartbreak of a midwife?
> —Sister MorningStar, CPM, Midwestern U.S.

The nature of homebirth midwifery care means that the client and her midwives build an intensely personal relationship that is unusual in the professional world. The goal of midwives is to provide safe, healthy, and empowering care to families through the childbearing year. The route to attaining that goal requires a gradual layering of mutual trust, open communication, comfort, and understanding. Many midwives have found that after serving a woman through her pregnancy and birth, the bonding experience gives way to a lasting friendship. Unlike other business relationships where necessary barriers exist between the professional and the client, midwives are required to make those intimate connections as part of their everyday work.

Elizabeth Davis, midwife and author, explains the hormonal basis behind the mother-midwife bond: "When a mother is releasing high levels of oxytocin, and the midwife is following the mother's lead, the midwife will actually entrain with the mother. This means that the mother's energy will influence and shape the midwife's experience. With entrainment, deep bonding also occurs. For some women, especially if they have not had a good relationship with their mother, the relationship with their midwife may be the deepest bond they have ever known."

Because of this strong bond, midwives may experience elation when the birth is triumphant for the mother or satisfaction when she helps the mother overcome an obstacle in her birth. Although midwives know that the outcomes of births are unpredictable, the midwife herself may feel emotionally invested in the mother having a satisfying birth at home.

> If you have a sense of gentle birth in your own heart, as a provider you will find a way for that family. You keep eye contact with gentle touches, you keep that humility, you keep praying. You also know darn well that you'll never be able to understand what they're going through.
> —Katherine Bradshaw, CPM, Northeastern U.S.

> I have a personal relationship with my midwife and she was so excited to come to my house in labor—we both had an attachment to my beautiful homebirth. When I transferred, she was pretty sad. She wanted me to give birth at home.
> —Maia (2012/HBC, Western U.S.)

> We had a moment where I could see in her eyes that my heartbreak was her heartbreak. She knew how badly I wanted something else and we were sharing the grief of that loss together.
> —Ann (2011/HBC, Midwestern U.S.)

Over the course of prenatal care, midwives build an intimate relationship with the mother and gain insight into her relationships, her work and home life, her fears, and her hopes. They may see each other socially and have common acquaintances in the community. When this client has a homebirth cesarean, the midwife may feel disappointment for her and her baby, and if she has connections with the woman outside of midwifery, she may feel a heavier sense of obligation and commitment to serving her well.

The personal life of the midwife

Not only does the midwife enjoy getting to know the woman, her partner, and her family, but sometimes the client begins to see her midwife as an ordinary woman outside of the office, with a family, hobbies, and life challenges. In many professions there is a distinct line between professional conduct at work and an individual's personal life. For midwives, the lines often blur between professional and personal, especially due to the hours and familiarity involved in caring for women who are pregnant, birthing, and newly mothering.

In some cases, a midwife giving insight into her personal life can enrich the bond between her and the mother. A midwife may welcome a worried mother into her home as she is finishing her dinner, just to check the baby's heartbeat. She may stop by a client's home with her own baby in tow to drop off the birth tub. As the client begins to learn more about her midwife, she may find that their shared connections and interests help them build a stronger relationship.

On a different occasion, the midwife might reveal that she was up for two nights caring for her sick grandmother so she's requesting a later appointment time for a visit. Giving clients simple explanations regarding personal issues if it affects their care is not only appropriate, it can also help the client understand that her midwife isn't neglecting or mistreating her. This is even more important when care taking HBC clients, who might already feel emotionally bruised and vulnerable.

The challenge for midwives is to walk the line between appropriately divulging personal details and considering the client's emotional and mental needs. Midwives want to protect a woman's emotional space and not drag in unnecessary information that would distract her, make her feel shame, or shift the focus away from her and her needs. It can help clients to see that midwives truly care about them and strive to be with them whenever they need, but they are also individuals with complex lives. When there are opportunities to build a solid two-way relationship between the mother and her midwife, the result is a deeper connection and better experience for both.

The rewards of serving HBC women

Midwives are sometimes surprised to find that in light of a challenging cesarean birth, their relationship with their clients are strengthened, communication is open and honest, or families now regard them as close friends or mentors. The challenges for midwives serving HBC families are complex, but the rewards can provide deep emotional or spiritual satisfaction. Sometimes, these rewards are immediate, like witnessing a moment of utter bliss when the mother first kisses or nurses her baby after surgery. Perhaps the midwife listens to the woman's partner share his heart-felt gratitude for the time she spent supporting the couple in labor. The midwife may get to hold a baby while the exhausted mother sleeps, and sometimes the midwife will enjoy sharing a meal with the family months after the birth. These moments of satisfaction are not exclusive to the HBC experience, but for a midwife who supported a family through a difficult homebirth cesarean, the simple rewards are even sweeter.

Because of the extensive level of care and interaction she has with her clients, every birth offers a midwife opportunities to gain knowledge and wisdom, but HBCs hold even more potential to enrich the midwife's perspective. Sometimes, these nuggets of insight are very apparent; other times the lessons are oblique and can only be seen with the gifts of time and distance. A new midwife may learn that her comment intended to soothe a grieving mother about her potential for a VBAC was misguided and hurtful to the mother. She will understand how to be more sensitive in the future and might simply sit attentively, while the grieving mother processes her feelings about her birth.

Serving women with pre-labor HBCs

Sometimes, a midwife supports a client through an HBC prior to the onset of labor, for instance when the client's health status or baby's position makes even a vaginal birth in the hospital risky. In this case, there can be fewer negative interactions with hospital staff, who may instead praise the midwife for "doing the right thing" by bringing the mother to the hospital. Deep inside, she might feel like a traitor, transporting a client who fears the hospital into the environment she most wanted to avoid. While she may have the gift of time and good rapport with the attending physician, the midwife can still suffer from feelings of powerlessness and lack of control in the hospital setting. Or she may feel like she relinquishes her integrity, speaking guardedly to the one nurse who has terrible homebirth "train wreck" stories, in order to keep peace in the room. The midwife cannot give her client the type of care she would like, and she cringes to see that despite her efforts to help the woman advocate for herself, interventions are done for the sake of expediency and routine.

Alternatively, these pre-labor HBCs can allow a midwife to give fantastic care to her client, resulting in a better birth experience and a strong mother-midwife bond throughout. When a midwife has time to help a woman prepare for what will happen during her hospital stay, and she can consult with a medical team who agree to provide compassionate care to the family, she can facilitate a smoother birth experience for the mother and baby.

> As far as I know, I was my midwife's first HBC and I believe it hit her hard. At the time of my daughter's birth, she had a 6-month old who had been born in the hospital after three days of labor at home. She could share my feelings on the loss of the homebirth. She gave me a shoulder on which to cry and as much information as I could process.
> —JAIME (2011/HBC, MIDWESTERN U.S.)

Communication with HBC clients

During interviews, midwives reported that when a birth is complicated, especially in a homebirth cesarean, clients are often unhappy with the care their birth team provided. Women and their partners may feel betrayed, disappointed, angry, or abandoned by their midwives. To the care provider who felt fondness and connection with her client, this sudden shift in the relationship can feel terribly distressing, and she may wonder how to continue to provide care while also addressing these uncomfortable conversations.

> When you've "done everything right," then that's all you can do. Watching a mom have to sign consent for surgery, even if she is making a fully informed decision, still rips my heart right out of my chest. Sometimes I cry the whole way home. Most often it helps to sift through everything with a trusted peer. But I know I can't control a birth outcome or a woman's perception of her birth experience.
> —MERIBETH GLENN, TRADITIONAL MIDWIFE, NORTHEASTERN U.S.

In some HBCs, the mother and midwife both recognize that the midwife "did all the right things" and that the baby still needed to be born by cesarean. The midwife may feel grateful for her intuition that prompted the transport, and she may have no lingering doubts about her role in attending the birth. If the mother has positive feelings about her midwifery care, the relationship can be especially satisfying for both the new mother and her midwife.

In many HBC situations, however, the midwife is challenged by both the outcome of the birth and the client's reactions to the care she provided. Midwife Lennon Clark struggled as a less experienced midwife when providing postpartum care for HBC mothers: "Sometimes I felt uneasy around the mom because she had a cesarean after we spent months talking about a homebirth. My inclination was to run away from her emotions and avoid talking about the birth. It wasn't out of malice, but it's distressing because the mom didn't get what she wanted. Now I feel like I've gotten better about addressing that."

Midwives sometimes continue to provide postpartum care without allowing full and honest conversations to unfold about how her care served the woman. The midwife may worry that unleashing a strong emotional re sponse will cause the new mother further pain. Or she may not recognize that inviting women to process their feelings about their care is an essential component in facilitating a sense of closure and healing after a difficult birth. This attempt to suppress the flood of emotions women feel after an HBC can feel safe for the midwife, who may be fearful of hearing how her care missed the mark or, worse yet, was negligent or harmful. The anticipation of hearing words of hurt and anger from a client can leave even a veteran midwife feeling scared, vulnerable, or defensive.

In cases where a new mother is satisfied with the care of her midwifery team, it can still be difficult to begin a conversation about the HBC because the midwife understands that the experience was painful for the mother and she herself may have unresolved feelings about her care.

I'm often at a loss for words when moms start sharing from a vulnerable place after a homebirth cesarean. Sometimes I find myself hoping that we don't have these difficult conversations.
—DEBBIE WONG, CPM, SOUTHERN U.S.

You cannot be afraid to talk to a mother—not for your own self and not for her. It's like after a loss or a death of any kind, the cultural default is to want to respect the mother's space and leave her alone. And that's where a lot of women feel abandoned. There's so much loss and disappointment after an HBC and people just don't know what to say or how to act.
—INGRID ANDERSSON, CNM, MIDWESTERN U.S.

The midwife may be hearing feedback from other support people who have their own opinions and emotions about how the birth turned out. The doula may want to call the midwife to discuss how she felt about the birth, or the mother's partner may want to share how angry she is at how the nurses treated the mother and baby. Not only is the midwife helping the mother come to terms with her birth outcome, she will often caretake the emotions of others involved in the HBC, helping them process their grief and providing perspective on how the birth unfolded. It can be helpful for the midwife to simply acknowledge the challenging nature of the birth and, when appropriate, share her own feelings of sadness or disappointment. She can also provide resources for therapy and grief counseling for those support people who are struggling to cope with the outcome of the birth. (See Appendix C, Resources for HBC Mothers and Families.)

The self-doubt and blame game
On the heels of serving a woman through an HBC, a midwife may wonder if she did everything right or if she missed a red flag along the way. In many HBC cases, the exact reasons for needing a cesarean are unclear, and this leaves room for conjecture by the mother, partner, birth team, hospital staff, and family. Feelings of self-doubt are common for midwives following a homebirth cesarean, and it can be hard for a midwife to reconcile her own feelings while still helping the new family work through their complex web of emotions.

I tell clients that I wonder what would have happened if I had done something different. I feel now like I can be more honest with women about my own curiosities. But it's easy to feel sad about how it happened.
—KORI PIENOVI, CNM, WESTERN U.S.

You feel bad and wonder if there's something else you could have done. You
have your own mourning about it.
—Heather Hack Sullivan, CPM, Western U.S.

It's hard for my midwife ego.
—Ellie Legare, CPM, Western U.S.

After an HBC, it's difficult for me to know if I did enough.
—Amanda Roe, naturopathic midwife, Western U.S.

Beyond wondering and self-reflection, sometimes midwives assume a level of guilt for how a birth unfolds and whether or not the cesarean could have been avoided. In describing an HBC she attended, Maggie Ogden, a nurse midwife, shared the following: "It was my fault for missing the breech. She had no choice when I said we needed to go to the hospital, and she trusted me. I feel really clear that I made a mistake, but when we learned of the baby's position in labor, I made the best recommendation I could at the time. I'm really sad and really sorry that it happened that way."

My midwives are humans, allowed to make mistakes, and their job is a difficult
one. I have played the blame game, blaming first myself, then God, then the
midwives.
—Carol (2012/HBC, Western U.S.)

Just as HBCs can deal a hard blow to a mother's ego, they can also leave midwives struggling to rebuild self-esteem and trust in their own professional capabilities. A midwife has concerns about how others will view her after an HBC, plus she feels layers of doubt, fear, and shame percolating deep within herself. A midwife might worry what her colleagues will think or say about her. She might perceive that some of the hospital staff are looking at her with disdain when she transports yet another client in need of a cesarean. A family member of hers might make an offhanded remark about her needing to quit midwifery and find a less stressful job. This layering of actual or perceived judgment can feed a midwife's festering sense of failure.

I go through a period of intense self-reflection and self-criticism because I
really want people to have a vaginal birth.
—Silke Akerson, CPM, Western U.S.

The midwife's ego

The sense of failure, self-doubt, and criticism are the shared domain of the mother and her birth team, yet often each is reluctant to initiate open conversation about this. According to midwife Heather Rische, "There is hesitancy among midwives to admit that they could have done something differently when their HBC clients come to them to process their birth stories. They might be afraid that their clients will get mad or spread rumors about their care."

Needing to strike the right balance of humility and self-confidence, midwives, like all working professionals, can sometimes allow their egos to interfere with providing good care to women. When a midwife's defeated self-image or her fears get in the way of her candid reflection with a client, she unwittingly blocks avenues for her own growth.

Imagine an exhausted mother sitting in her midwife's office weeks after her HBC. When she tries to initiate a conversation about the birth, the midwife's body language conveys that she is guarded or dismissive of the topic. Perhaps the midwife stares down at the chart in her lap instead of meeting the mother's eyes. She reassures the mother that the cesarean was necessary, the words spilling from her mouth in hopes that she need not reveal her own insecurities. Sensing the midwife's discomfort with talking about the birth, the mother's suspicions of personal failure are confirmed, and she sinks deeper into her own feelings of shame. The midwife has just demonstrated to her client that HBCs are so disgraceful that they must not be frankly discussed.

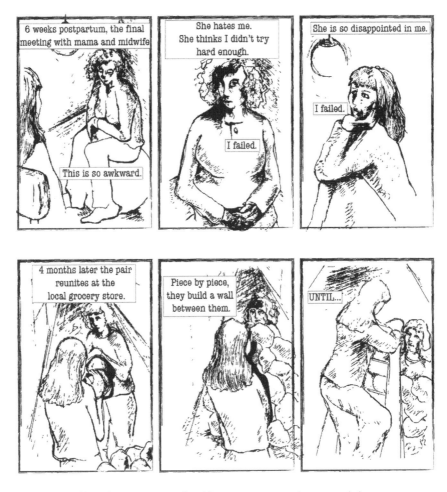

Midwife and Mom during an uncomfortable postpartum appointment and then an encounter outside the office.

Hartman, 2013

Women often choose the calling to become a midwife in the hope that they can give mothers holistic and unhurried care that is largely unavailable in the hospital. In addition, midwives sometimes witness insensitive, negligent, or poor care by the hospital staff. This can lead midwives to perceive that their care is superior to that given by hospital-based providers. Midwives may mistakenly believe that with good assessment skills, open communication, and a strong knowledge base, that they can prevent unwanted client outcomes, including homebirth cesarean, postpartum depression, or birth trauma. Midwives may neglect to screen, acknowledge, and provide support thinking that their care alone can ward off any negative fallout.

For new midwives, or midwives with limited experience in cesarean birth aftercare, it can be difficult to not only process feelings about the experience but it can be even harder if the midwife feels she is poorly equipped to assess the mental, emotional, and physical status of the new mother. Corinne Rupp, a midwife now studying to become a nurse midwife, says:

> As a new apprentice I remember feeling underprepared for postpartum visits with the mamas who gave birth surgically. I wish an experienced midwife had told me what to expect and what to do. Some women seemed shell-shocked; others seemed fine. In the early visits especially, I didn't know what to do to emotionally support them. I felt as lost and alone as the moms probably did. I didn't know how to make space for them to talk.

A midwife who feels emotionally vulnerable following an HBC might begin a conversation by seeking the mother's permission to share her own feelings. This allows the mother to choose to engage in the conversation or wait until she feels ready. The midwife can also maintain an open channel of communication by offering to touch base with her client in six months or a year, when both have had time to process the birth and may have insights to share with each other. For example, after an HBC where the midwife feels regret about not transporting a mother sooner, she might say something like, "I have some thoughts about how your transport and birth went. I'm wondering if at some point you would be interested in hearing my perceptions." In this case, the client is free to decline or accept or share that she is unsure at this point if she wants to hear her midwife's input.

Listening to feedback from clients

They want to love us, and they want to be thankful to us. And you do care about each other. For those reasons, I think it's probably really hard for women to give us feedback.
—Kori Pienovi, CNM, Western U.S.

Some of the midwives we interviewed have a process for seeking feedback from their HBC clients and integrating that feedback into their midwifery practice. This feedback can help to calibrate her own emotional responses and feelings about her care for the client. Requesting evaluation not only allows the client to speak her mind and voice her gratitude or frustrations, but it can give the midwife clarity and context for the relationship as they move forward.

Some midwives ask for feedback as the care progresses. Others set aside a specific time in the postpartum period for processing the birth and feedback. A few midwives solicit input on the client's experience using written feedback forms. Kori Pienovi offers that she sometimes says to clients: "You can write me a letter if there were things you were angry, upset, or curious about."

If the client is unhappy with the midwife's care or thinks that she made mistakes, the midwife may struggle to provide care for that client after the birth. Perhaps the partner is angry that the midwife didn't mention transport earlier or that she didn't do enough to prevent a cesarean. When the mother or partner is angry with the midwife, it can be uncomfortable to continue to provide care especially if they are unwilling to directly address their reasons for being dissatisfied.

> We had two midwives and I didn't give either of them feedback. I believe they were open to it, but I was so overwhelmed after the hospital that I never put any time or effort into connecting with them after the birth. I regret that now, but my energy was just sapped.
>
> Also, I didn't understand, really, what had happened. How do you give someone constructive criticism when you don't know where mistakes were made nor what could have been done differently?
> —Michael, partner of Serena (2009/HBC, Southern U.S.)

Returning to the client's home for a postpartum visit is fraught with emotions for the midwife if she perceives disapproval from the family. Pienovi says, "Sometimes I try to guess at what they might be feeling. 'I'm wondering if you might feel upset that I offered to break your water.' So I open it up for feedback." Soliciting critical feedback is not easy for many midwives, who want to please their clients and feel that they did a good job serving them. However, when they can view the evaluation process as an opportunity for growth and possibly repairing a broken relationship with the client, the benefits clearly outweigh the drawbacks for both the new mother and the midwife.

At other times, the midwife may sense that the client has negative thoughts about her role in the birth but may be afraid to ask the client directly. When the client, feeling tired and vulnerable, fails to express her anger or disappointment with the midwife and the midwife senses that withholding, it can become an uncomfortable dynamic that further prevents understanding and resolution.

> I'm having a hard time being honest with my midwife—I won't give her feedback. She cried because she feels like she messed up the birth of my baby and I don't have the heart to tell her that I'm unhappy with the way she handled things.
> —SKY (2008/HBC, NORTHEASTERN U.S.)

> I wonder if she just didn't want to face me.
> —TERRA (2011/HBC, NORTHEASTERN U.S.)

Midwife Silke Akerson explains how she approaches these situations: "I usually do it by stating some observation, and then saying, 'I've noticed since the cesarean you aren't talking about your feelings. I just want to let you know that I'm really comfortable with talking about your experience.' I've said to clients, 'I think up until the cesarean your experience has been really positive, and I know that you might be scared to let me know if you are disappointed and angry, and I want you to know that you can tell me.'"

> There is no right or wrong question to ask a mother. It's all about the attitude with which you ask. Are you truly open-hearted and of a quiet mind when you say to a mother, 'Is there anything you wish I had done differently?'
> I can feel the difference when someone's mind is quiet and their heart is open versus someone who is armored and really doesn't want to listen. We understand that mothers go on to raise their families, midwives go on to catch another baby, and doulas go on to sit at another birth. Empowering women to get their truth on the table is good for all of us.
> —ELIZABETH DAVIS, CPM AND AUTHOR, WESTERN U.S.

Setting boundaries

Following an HBC, clients may express strong negative feelings about the care they received, and it can be hard for midwives to be clear on how they should internalize these feelings. Akerson describes the need for midwives to clarify their own boundaries. "I think midwives take too much responsibility and have poor boundaries. There's a big difference between saying 'I am really open to hearing what you have to say' and 'I'm willing to take responsibility for what you have to say.' In the case of a cesarean that involves trauma, women can sometimes direct their anger at their midwife because she is a safe person, while they wouldn't feel comfortable raging at their doctor. It's really important for midwives to differentiate between what they can take responsibility for and what they can't."

In some cases, a midwife may feel blindsided by her client's anger at her or feel it is unjustified. When this happens, the gift of understanding and perspective can help a midwife moderate her own defensive reaction. Renowned birth professional Penny Simkin explains one way for birth workers to handle a client's anger:

> You can say to yourself that she has very good reasons for feeling angry and reacting this way. You may be the target right now, but you are not the reason. If her perception is that your care was lacking, she is right to feel that way. She is angry because of other things in her life that have led to that. You can empathize, telling her you recognize how awful she feels, and that you feel badly for what happened to her. When she feels she's heard, that may be the first step in her recognizing that you were there with her. You may be able to get her to soften a little if she doesn't feel any push back or silence from you.

This ability to set aside one's ego, and listen and empathize with an angry client, is essential to rebuilding broken relationships and concluding care with a sense of resolution.

Occasionally, a family may reject the continued care from their midwife and may or may not explain why, leaving the midwife to ponder reasons. Midwife Lennon Clark shared an occasion where, despite her efforts to maintain contact with an HBC client, the mother didn't return her calls. "I have a lot of unsettled feelings around that birth. I wonder why she cut off contact with me." In these cases, the midwife may never have an opportunity to hear the client's intentions and feelings, and that can be uncomfortable for a midwife who seeks clarity and understanding in her relationships. On the part of the client, she may never feel like she was able to voice her frustrations, and that can prevent her from finding peace in her experience.

Seeking emotional support and perspective from another midwife can be a key to resolutely navigating all births that a midwife attends. When an HBC occurs, the midwife is left to reconcile her own feelings of disappointment or grief, and she may carry these emotions with her into the next client's birth.

Vicarious trauma

If the HBC was traumatic for the mother, the midwife may suffer trauma as well. According to the Headington Institute, which promotes psychological wellbeing for humanitarian workers in disaster relief areas, "Vicarious trauma is the process of change that happens because you care about other people who have been hurt, and feel committed or responsible to help them. When you identify with the pain of people who have endured terrible things, you bring their grief, fear, anger, and despair into your own awareness and experience. Over time this process can lead to changes in your psychological, physical, and spiritual well-being.[13]"

> When you go to a birth, you are always carrying two bags. In one hand you have your equipment bag. In your other hand you carry an invisible bag holding your biases, expectations, and emotional challenges in your personal life. You will always have that invisible bag, but when you walk through the door to attend a birthing woman, you've got to know what's in it.
> —ELIZABETH DAVIS, CPM AND AUTHOR, WESTERN U.S.

HBCs and the birth professional community

When a midwife serves a family through an HBC, she might not only self-reflect on the care that she gave, but she may find that others in her professional community are questioning her choices. Other midwives and the hospital staff may be searching for answers or assigning "blame" for the homebirth cesarean, so a midwife may feel compelled to defend her actions and deal with the unanswered questions. She will often need to peer review

---

13   Pearlman, L. A. & McKay, L. (2008). Headington Institute: *Online Training Module Four: Understanding and Addressing Vicarious Trauma.* Retrieved September 22, 2014 from http://www.headington-institute.org/files/vtmoduletemplate2_ready_v2_85791.pdf

the birth with midwives, who will express a variety of opinions on how she cared for her client. Even when she follows the accepted community standards and works within mandated risk criteria, she may be asked to justify her actions, which she fears could reveal perceived inexperience, lack of skill, or even poor judgment.

> At the time, the whole area where I lived was unfriendly to VBACs, especially homebirth VBACs. In the hospital I could hear the doctors tearing into my midwife about why she took me on as a client. She was attacked. She left the hospital and never came back. I understand her situation, but I felt a little dumped by her.
> —TARA (1999/HOSPITAL BIRTH, 2006/CS, 2008, 2010/HBC; WESTERN U.S.)

While a midwife's primary obligation is her clients, she also values the approval and support of her fellow midwives. For those practicing in isolated areas or states where midwifery is illegal, the relative lack of a local midwifery community means that some midwives will find no opportunity to review and process difficult homebirth cesareans. In addition, strained relations between the medical and midwifery communities can compound a midwife's stress following an HBC.

> I know in some areas there is a lot of tension between midwives and hospitals. My midwife brought that tension to the hospital. But the hospital took the higher road. They were awesome and very sympathetic about the transport.
> —JUSTIN, PARTNER OF TERRA (2012/HBC, NORTHEASTERN U.S.)

Because the homebirth midwife has transparency in her care, midwives may perceive that there is a diffusion of accountability for staff within a hospital setting since medical tasks are fulfilled by many different providers. Since a homebirth midwife is not surrounded by a large staff but is solely accountable for her actions in caring for her clients, she cannot blame a mistake on an inexperienced nurse or an error in the pharmacy. This transparency and responsibility can lead to a feeling of vulnerability that can be scary if the local political climate is unsupportive of homebirth midwives.

Following any birth outcome that was unwanted, including a homebirth cesarean, a client may initiate legal action against her midwife, or the midwife may be targeted by the hospital, investigated by the licensing board, or even by law enforcement officials. Homebirth midwives in most states do not carry malpractice insurance, and so the additional stress from the financial threat of lawsuits can encourage a sense of self-protection and defensiveness.

When a client has an HBC and the midwife worries that she might be professionally sanctioned as a result, the care that she gives her clients can be interlaced with her worries and additional stresses. In some cases, the clients may terminate their care with her, or they may rally to her defense and strengthen the bond they have built. Either way, the midwife will need to galvanize her own support network and draw upon the strength of compassionate peers, family, and friends who can sustain her during this stressful time.

Another layer of challenge for midwives is birth gossip that can undermine her reputation and even mean a loss of business. Midwives are bound by codes of confidentiality and understand that sharing intimate details of a client's birth is not only unprofessional and illegal but could be a devastating invasion of a family's privacy.

In cases where the information shared about the midwife is positive, it can serve as a powerful endorsement of her care and skills. But when the information is negative or erroneous, it can undermine a midwife's reputation. In such cases, the midwife herself may not have the opportunity to clarify details of the birth or share her perspective, since she must maintain confidentiality about the client's case.

Keeping the home fires burning

Leaving a new mother resting in the hospital after an HBC, a midwife looks forward to returning home for sleep, food, and to reconnecting with her family or friends. The mental shift from caring for a client to self-care, tending to children, or fulfilling other personal or professional obligations can be stressful when the midwife has not had adequate sleep or nourishment.

One of the biggest challenges for a midwife on the heels of a long HBC is the level of fatigue she experiences both during and after the birth. During a transport, the midwife needs to present herself in a professional manner, share the client's pertinent medical chart information, and help advocate for the needs and desires of the family. Heather Hack notes that walking into the hospital with a client, "you are exhausted, and you have to be even more pulled-together. It would be nice if you could have new clothes and a shower, but that doesn't happen. You're trying to be professional, ask questions, and be their advocate in the middle of this. It's really tricky."

Ideally, the midwife returns home to a warm bed, a silent phone, and a sympathetic family so she can recoup the sleep she has lost. In reality, returning home often means a quick nap and then a full day of prenatal visits or family commitments. Not only must a midwife mask her exhaustion with caffeine, a shower, or sheer force of will, she needs to shift into caregiving mode for her family once more.

> *The long births I attended during my first years were hard on my kids—they were so extremely shuffled around. They never knew who would be there when they woke up. But they knew when I was there, I'd be unconditionally loving, even when I hadn't slept in two nights and was grieving the loss of a vaginal birth for a woman I'd served for days. I'd calculate how long I'd been gone— guilt-ridden and deeply contemplating why service to other families was more important than my own. It didn't make any sense, yet it made complete and total sense. The way my love is spread between my clients and my own children is a bit like doing drugs. There is a compulsion to keep doing more, though there is pain and suffering as a result.*
>
> *I'm used to coming home from long, grueling births and not being able to sleep because of my kids' needs. I'd feel a simmering level of anxiety about all the tasks at hand, until something gave. Often it was anger, out of frustration. Other times it was sadness, out of devastation—the kind one only reaches when in the most piercing emotional crisis, or when extremely sleep-deprived.*
>
> *I was also forever in debt to my family members who pulled off my kids' birthday parties in my absence. Sometimes I felt huge guilt for what I'd set them up to do. I felt a deeper sense of pride, however, for being the kick-ass mom I was to have made a plan B strong enough to withstand my absence.*
> —MELISSA GORDON-MAGNUS, CPM, WESTERN U.S.

While the midwife herself gains spiritual or emotional satisfaction from fulfilling her duty and seeing women through the process of an HBC, her family only knows that they have been missing her. As a result, she often feels guilty for being away from them and needs to establish her own balance of obligations in order to thrive in her work. She might do this by limiting the number of births she attends, calling an apprentice or other midwife to temporarily provide care for the new mother, or making a date to spend uninterrupted time with her partner or children once she has rested.

An additional layer of challenge following an HBC is the financial strain some midwives experience. When a midwife transports a client, health insurance providers only reimburse for care at the location of the actual birth. This means that the midwife has essentially provided extensive care for a client on an unpaid basis. Midwives accept that this is how the insurance industry operates, and they are hopeful that they can bill for some portion of the prenatal care they provided. However, it can be a stretch to absorb the cost of care for clients who often need extra home visits, extra phone time, and extra support. When a client pays out-of-pocket, she can feel pinched for money when paying the midwife's fees, and then having a hefty hospital birth bill to deal with as well. In these cases, the midwife's fees may go unpaid.

This financial hardship can cause relationship tension in a family. When a midwife's partner has had to leave work early two days in a row and pay the babysitter for extended hours, the lack of payment for a cesarean birth can be a bitter pill to swallow.

> Years ago, I added more stress by letting my emotions come forward when I'd been calculating how much time and money had been lost while she was at a homebirth cesarean. Then I saw how tired and burned out she was returning from these births, and that she just needed me to welcome her back home again. Now I try to be supportive because this is just what our family is.
> —ROBERT, PARTNER OF LAURIE PERRON MEDNICK, CPM, WESTERN U.S.

Recharging the batteries

After an emotionally exhausting birth, some midwives have routine ways of caring for themselves. These self-care rituals allow the midwife to make the transition from caring for another woman to caring for herself, while also leaving space for processing the birth experience as the healthcare provider. Some midwives will ask a colleague to provide back-up care for clients so that they can rest and reconnect with family. Other midwives will take a long bath, spend time in the garden, or relax with a book. One midwife finds that eating eggs from her own hens is grounding and nourishing, while another midwife exercises to keep her body resilient and healthy.

> My self-care includes regular massages and pedicures.
> —MELISSA GORDON-MAGNUS, CPM, WESTERN U.S.

> As a midwife, I take care of myself by making sure the mom has everything in place: someone who can watch the children, be the guardian of the door, make food, and do laundry.
> —SISTER MORNINGSTAR, CPM, MIDWESTERN U.S.

When midwives attend birth after birth without seeking renewal and self-care, not only is it more difficult to be fully present for subsequent births, but it can lead to burnout. Over time, the cumulative effect of attending challenging births can be difficult for a midwife and other members of her team. According to psychotherapist Karen Jackson Forbes, "Burnout is partly not having some way of understanding things that didn't go right. They might be blaming themselves for things they did or didn't do. Even if there is nothing they did wrong, it's a *this happened on my watch* kind of feeling." This cumulative sense of burnout can be exacerbated when the midwife has no closure with a family who experienced a traumatic HBC, and the birth can remain an open wound that never quite heals, both for the family and the midwife. In some cases, midwives will seek therapy to help process deep layers of grief and to provide a fresh slate for moving forward in their work.

> With this work comes the need for good boundaries and emotional release. I've learned to recognize where my emotional, physical, and spiritual boundaries are, and when I'm carrying the energy of others in my field. I make choices about removing those energies for the purpose of my own well-being and healing, and in order to be fully available to each of my clients.
> —ELIZABETH DAVIS, CPM AND AUTHOR, WESTERN U.S.

> We sit in intensity in people's lives over and over again. If we keep going from one birth to the next, we are bringing the dregs of what happened before to the current birth. So I try to sit with my partner or apprentice to debrief as soon after the birth as possible. We talk about what feelings came up, what worked for us in our support or if the support was too thin, how to make the

next situation better. Each person gets to debrief what her perception was and what could have been different. And that really helps us to show up fresh for the next one.
—MARY JACKSON, RN, LM; WESTERN U.S.

Midwifery is a job unlike any other. It requires technical skills and a deep knowledge of birth, and it demands that midwives open their hearts to a steady stream of relationships with women who entrust them with their lives. When a client has an HBC, her midwife has her own separate but interconnected feelings and perceptions about the birth and the care that she provided the family. If she can work through these complex emotions while simultaneously assisting the new mother in her own healing process, the experience can be gratifying for the midwife, who learns more with each woman she serves.

Birth Story: Without Ceremony, a Tragedy Dangles

—A Conversation with Dave, an HBC Father

Q: What happened when you realized Courtney might need to transport to the hospital?

A: I understand how emotionally fragile a laboring mother can be, but I wanted to talk about the hospital an hour before anyone else did. I brought it up to one of our midwives and she shut me down saying we weren't ready to have that conversation. But I was ready. I wasn't heard in that situation and I was only trying to mentally and emotionally prepare myself so things would have been more strategic and less dire for me.

Once transport was decided, the way we were keeping track of time changed and that's where Courtney got lost in the process. Before transport, time was like an old-fashioned pocket watch; and after deciding to leave it became a digital clock tracking to the tenths of seconds. Once I knew we were going to the hospital, I forgot about Courtney being in labor, so I was surprised every time she had a contraction. It was a head trip because all of a sudden the real world was invading our sacred space.

Q: What would you have done to internally ready yourself to transport if you had been given the time?

A: I would have slowed down and not gotten sucked into the frantic energy of doing things and wondering how we were going to get to the hospital. I would have given myself a minute and said, "Okay, she's not going to die, the baby is not going to die, you're okay, she's okay. Just get a hold of yourself and don't be so dark." I would have given myself a pep talk. What I needed was slow, quiet breathing, but there was no space offered for that.

Q: What was it like for you to step into the hospital?

A: There is a romantic component to homebirth—it's like selling a person on a wedding—you expect the candles and soft music and we were prepared for that situation. The hospital was a huge shock to my system. Neither Courtney nor I were engaged with her labor once there, and I was no longer engaged with my own experience. I was a zombie; my brain had been eaten but my body was still moving.

Q: What happened when you were separated from her while she was being prepped for surgery?

A: One of the midwives rubbed my back and that touch was really important for me because I was so distraught. I broke down crying. I wondered what a cesarean would do to Courtney. I knew she'd heal physically, but I wasn't sure if she would emotionally make it.

Q: What was the hospital stay like for you?

A: In a way, because Courtney was treated with so much respect, our stay there shielded us from what was to come, and I'm grateful for that. The nurses joked with me about typical stuff: "Oh, you'll have to change diapers now." But no one pulled me aside and said, "Just so you know, your wife may be a basket case. She may get suicidal at some point. So you'd better know what to do." And four months later Courtney was suicidal. Things got pretty grave.

Q: How did you support your new family during those first weeks?

A: Even though our daughter was seven pounds of helplessness with spindly legs that flopped over her ears, I felt more driven to support Courtney. I felt like anything I could do to create space for her was worth doing. But two months in, I'd already started to move on from the birth and I wanted Courtney to do the same. Instead, she was dipping further down into postpartum depression.

This was a difficult stretch for our relationship because I was able to partition things, but for her everything was a trigger to the birth. Not being able to make breast milk, in my mind, was not being able to make milk. For Courtney, not being able to make milk led right back to the fact that she'd had a cesarean. Even small things were apt to cause violent and angry reactions. If I took certain things for what they were—if I didn't understand how everything was linked in her mind—then I could get the sense that it was crazy for her to feel that way.

It took me a while to come around to her perspective. I know Courtney was certain she was explaining herself correctly, and that she thought I should understand. But by now, in the second and third months, I wanted to go back to life "as usual." When she told me she was tired and alone, I wasn't hearing that she was scared and depressed. She wanted me to see all the connections, but I didn't know that was what she wanted. In a way, she hadn't found the vocabulary to communicate what was going on. That would come later with therapy.

It was around this time that I started to fall into my own postpartum depression. The adrenaline was gone, and I looked around one day and wondered where my own support was. I felt very desperate and alone quite often, and I didn't have anyone to turn to.

None of my friends could relate to my situation. Even the ones that I was able to connect with, people who were compassionate by nature, couldn't relate. They'd understand our situation in general, but then I'd keep going on about all of the issues surrounding the birth and the postpartum, and their understanding seemed to just stop.

I did find help in strange places. Working with kids, for instance—their energy was great to be around. I also shared my experience with certain women in the workshops I teach. I never wanted to burden them, but they always wanted to hear our story. And, in a way, my sharing seemed to open up channels for their own sharing, even women whose children were in their teens and early 20s. It was as if they had closed a door on their own birth experiences before it was time, and now they had an opportunity to nudge it open a bit. So the healing went both ways.

Q: What kind of support did you need from your midwives?

A: Our midwives were available to a degree, but there was definitely a level of breaking off. When I realized that they weren't going to be paid because insurance was covering the hospital and not them, it played in my head. Why wouldn't they leave? How much time could they spend without getting paid? I always wondered how much more we would see of them.

We were thrust into finding our own support: lactation, milk sharing, hospital, hip doctors, therapy—our needs were all over the place. What we really needed was someone to mother Courtney, a compassionate third person to spend a few hours a day with her who didn't require us to bring her up to speed, someone who just knew how to care for her.

Q: What would have helped you heal from the birth experience?

A: Without ceremony, a tragedy dangles. People are afraid that talking about hurts will open old wounds. But those wounds are always open, and talking about them helps to soothe them. I wish very much that we had gotten together with our midwives to talk about what had happened. Just for a meal or something casual, not a regular appointment. And rather than avoid the elephant in the room and coo at the baby, we could have talked about our reality together.

Our midwives should have started this conversation. Courtney was in no state to do this, and they are the professionals. I would want them to be candid and open, and to come as listeners who were there to frame healing around ceremony. For me, four weeks would have been a good time for that to happen. After four weeks I started to move into other areas of my life and responsibilities. I started to move toward Lazadae more.

Q: Where are you now, 28 months after the birth?

A: I know that Courtney will always carry her scar. Seeing how triggered she sometimes can be tells me that the birth will stay with her. And I'm sensitive to that. I'm very quick to defend her right to still be processing things.

The HBC project has helped me become more understanding and sensitive to this, because it's not just a Courtney thing. The trauma around HBC is a global issue. It's very powerful, very moving, and very sad. Society doesn't want women to dwell and hurt; it just wants women to move forward, be moms, and get over it.

I feel like Courtney needs an annual day of ceremony that is about her and her body, not about Lazadae, and not even about the birth. Maybe she sets aside the day before the birth as the end of her dream, the end of her unscarred body. Because she really deserves a day that is separate from the actual birth.

Chapter 9

Wired for love:
caring for our babies as they grow

Written By: Claudia Baskind

Mothers who have unexpected or complicated events in birth tend to worry that their baby's life is ruined if they didn't have an initial bonding contact. That sense of worry about the bond is evidence of the bond itself. When women are concerned whether their bond is now jeopardized, if they've done all the right things, or if their babies are bonding, it's because the potential bond coming from their end is so strong. Their concern is a good sign.

Babies are best at one particular emotion when they're born, and that's love. They are wired for love. The need for a baby to bond with someone who will take care of him is so paramount that nothing can get in the way.

And when we acknowledge the wonderful things mothers do for their babies, we foster healing for everyone. Mothers need to hear that bonding doesn't always come naturally at first. It takes time.

—CAROL GRAY, CRANIOSACRAL THERAPIST AND RETIRED MIDWIFE, WESTERN U.S.

The natural birth movement vocally champions the benefits of drug-free childbirth, and our society tends to blame mothers for their children's challenges. These factors can easily lead an HBC mother to cultivate self-blame for her baby's birth experience and fear for her child's well-being as a result of her cesarean birth. Yet it is the cultivation of support for mothers and their own healing that in turn helps their babies be well after a difficult birth. Though many birth interventions can interfere with initial mother-child contact, there are ways to overcome these challenges.

This chapter urges a consideration that birth is neither the deciding event of a person's life nor the predictor of a person's life to come. Rather, birth is a hugely influential and significant event in a life that is already underway. Bonding happens prenatally and throughout the entire relationship of a

parent and child. When birth doesn't go as intended, as with homebirth cesarean, there are numerous ways to mitigate any potentially negative effects
and to strengthen the mother-child bond.

Beyond the birth

Prenatally, many HBC mothers we interviewed heard and read of potentially negative outcomes often associated with cesarean birth. These outcomes range quite broadly: bonding issues, digestive health problems, respiratory complications, autism, sensory processing disorders, emotional
and behavioral issues, and a tendency towards violence. Mothers we interviewed referred to a number of sources that influenced their beliefs about
the potential harm to babies of cesarean birth, including well-known natural birthing books, birth movies, blogs, childbirth education classes, birth
and health professionals, and family and friends. For an HBC mother, it
can be daunting to shift those acquired beliefs, trust that her baby is okay,
and genuinely believe that she will be able to provide the necessary care
should actual issues arise.

> I really hate what people say about cesarean babies being damaged or that
> they have emotional issues from how they were born. Birth would've been a
> hell of a ride however my son came out. Hearing all of the illnesses and con-
> ditions that are supposedly caused by cesarean birth really added a layer of
> meaningless and unnecessary guilt.
> —TRACY (2012/HBC, SOUTHERN U.S.)

> In response to my saying that I birthed with violence, I needed someone to
> tell me that such thinking was bullshit. My belief didn't begin to get unstuck
> until I was in a postpartum depression group and you couldn't tell who had
> birthed in what ways.
> —ANN (2011/HBC, MIDWESTERN U.S.)

Michel Odent, MD, retired obstetrician and international champion of
women's birthing rights, says that focusing purely on the birth event itself
provides too limited a view on the baby's whole development. He founded
the Primal Health Research Center in 1986 with the objective to test the
assumption that human health is shaped during the *primal period*, which
includes time *in utero*, birth, and the year following birth. The Primal
Health Database, says Odent, "is the only database specialized in studies

exploring the long-term consequences of what happens at the beginning of our life. Until now, the natural childbirth movement has only seen the short-term."

For HBC mothers steeped in the natural childbirth movement, problems arise when they begin to blame the mode of birth itself. Mothers develop a sense of guilt for their child's health issues or imagine possible concerns that may not exist. David Carroll, MD, a pediatrician who focuses on natural approaches for childhood health, states that in his practice he has only seen three characteristics common to cesarean-born children: a less molded head shape than babies born vaginally, more initial respiratory issues, and differences in gut flora. He emphasizes that these are correlations only and that it is inherently problematic to try to prove that a cesarean mode of birth is responsible for later-identified health issues:

> I see kids with many kinds of problems, such as speech or global developmental delays, with or without a cesarean. But are the two related? My guess is probably not. There are studies citing a higher rate of cesarean birth for kids who have autism, but there are multiple reasons why that can get confusing. Let's say that children with developmental delay or poor motor coordination have something different in their muscle tone or musculature that makes it harder for them to come out of the birth canal, and that makes them more likely to need a cesarean. Maybe the reason they had a cesarean had something to do with what caused the problem. In other words, the cesarean was a consequence of the existing problem. There is no valid data; it's all speculation. A lot of what you do after birth can have as much, if not greater impact on health, than how the birth happened.

Talking to baby

Many HBC mothers report feeling in deep connection and communication with their baby during pregnancy and labor, followed by a loss of connection in the time preceding the surgery, during the birth itself, or afterwards. One of the primary supports an HBC mother can provide to her baby after birth is to talk to him and explain what happened.

According to midwife and craniosacral therapist Mary Jackson, it is important that "the mother talk to her baby about the birth, to let baby know what her intentions were, and to tell baby that what she wanted was really different than what happened." Jackson recommends a mother offer "an apology around wherever her heart was broken." She offers this example: "I didn't want you to go away from me. While they were repairing me, you had to go the nursery and your dad went with you. I wanted to be with you in the worst way, and I'm sorry I wasn't able to do that."

Jackson explains what may happen after a cesarean birth:

> When the baby returns to mom, everybody expects a happy reunion but the baby may have big feelings to express before he can go to the breast and nurse. Mom may think that the baby doesn't like her if the baby settles down with dad but not her. The mother then has a bigger feeling of inadequacy—not only didn't she birth vaginally, but she can't soothe her baby. It's really important for the dad to give space so the mother and baby can work through their experience. Let mom hold the baby so they arrive together at a settled place.

> Later on, the mother's support person can slow things down for her as she tells the birth story to her baby: "And then there was the ride down the hall, and then the operating room, and the shaving." Slow it down as she tells the story, because her nervous system is re-experiencing these events.

As the mother tells the birth story, a listener can use touch (one of the four points of centering introduced in Chapter 3) and ask, "May I put my hand on your foot as you talk?" Whatever a mother feels disappointed about, a support person can find a way to include that in the present moment of storytelling for the mother and the baby. The mother can say, for example, "I couldn't be with you then, but I can be with you now, and you are nursing, and this is what I so wanted to do after the birth, and I'm so glad we are together now." This storytelling approach can be both a crucial first step and an ongoing support for a baby's healing and bonding.

When my daughter was little, I talked to her and apologized for how things happened. I explained that my sadness had nothing to do with her. Well before she could understand what I was saying, I felt like she could understand the intent.
—STEPHANIE (2008, 2012/HBC; NORTHEASTERN U.S.)

I received energetic work, often while breastfeeding, and the practitioner talked with her, verbalizing messages she was picking up from her body language: "I know that was hard. Oh, you were scared when you got here." After these sessions I had big emotional releases and felt more grounded. We also saw changes like better eye tracking and freer movement in her spine and hips.
—Courtney (2011/HBC, Western U.S.)

Have a bacterial perspective

For mothers, talking to and feeding their newborns is their primary focus. However, it can be difficult for an HBC mother to believe her baby is okay, or to bond with her baby when he is "colicky" or shows other signs of distress around feeding or digesting. Newborn gut health is one of the early challenges many HBC mothers need to navigate.

An HBC baby may face multiple obstacles to developing healthy gut flora, an important part of long-term digestive, immune, and overall health. It's worth noting that babies born vaginally in the hospital face some of these challenges as well. They may have trouble developing good gut health due to interference with the preservation of the baby's healthy bacteria or the transfer of the mother's bacteria to the baby, as well as the introduction of unhealthy bacteria from the hospital environment into the baby's system.

IV antibiotics, initial contact from people other than the parents, exposure to pathogens, and feeding interventions can all contribute to this challenge. In addition to the roadblocks for all hospital-born babies, a cesarean-born baby, depending on his station at the time of delivery, most likely is not exposed to the mother's vaginal secretions or fecal flora. He may then be immediately bathed, having most amniotic fluid, blood, vernix, and flora removed. If IV antibiotics are administered to the mother during labor or during surgery before cord-clamping, as is the standard U.S. hospital protocol, the baby may receive a direct dose of antibiotics that can skew his flora. Prenatally, providers can discuss the use of antibiotics and mothers can learn their choice points to make informed decisions.

I was given penicillin to empirically cover for Group Beta Strep since I declined the prenatal test and then was given Ancef in the OR. I assume I received three doses total, as that's the industry standard. But I only know about this because I read my medical records. I was never told I was getting antibiotics or what they were for.
—KRISTEN (2012/HBC, NORTHEASTERN U.S.)

In ideal circumstances during a cesarean birth, the baby is placed immediately on mom's chest. Cara Hafner, registered nurse and lactation consultant, emphasizes preserving a baby's flora by not bathing after birth. If blood, vernix, and amniotic fluid remain on the baby, he will ingest flora from his own hands; if there is skin-to-skin contact, the baby will also ingest flora that transfers from his mother's breasts and skin while feeding. Michel Odent notes the following:

> The first microbes that occupy the territory will become the rulers of the territory. The question is: who is the best person, from a bacterial perspective, to hold the baby? If there is co-habitation between the mother and the partner, then the partner can hold the baby. If they sleep and eat together, they have the same microbial world. This is, of course, if mom can't hold the baby.

Passing flora to baby

HBC mothers we interviewed were particularly aware of the benefits of passing healthy flora to their babies. Considering that a mother's flora can be altered by antibiotics during or prior to surgery, many mothers have—after the fact—wondered about the efficacy of preserving a vaginal swab collected before the birth to later colonize their babies orally or topically.

While many wish they had done this, none of the mothers we interviewed had. At the time of publication of this book, a study has been underway in Puerto Rico examining the effects of vaginal swabs on newborns, but there is inconclusive evidence about the effectiveness and the safety of such a practice.[14] David Carroll, MD offers that a post c-section vaginal

---

14   Dominguez-Bello, M. et al. *Proceedings of the National Academy of Sciences of the United States of America*, 24 May 2010. Mar. 2014.http://www.pnas.org/content/107/26/11971. full.pdf+html

swab may have no effect, as the mother's flora is immediately disrupted upon administration of IV antibiotics.

Mothers who are interested in using a vaginal swab preserved from before the birth to colonize their babies after birth may speak with their midwives about the benefits, risks, and safest methods of collecting, storing, and using a swab.

Naturopath and midwife Amanda Roe suggests that, after labors or births where antibiotics were administered, mothers can insert probiotics into their vaginas, as close to the cervix as possible, three times a day for ten days. On day five of this protocol, they can insert a finger into their vagina one to three times that day and inoculate the baby orally by putting that finger immediately in the baby's mouth to stimulate the sucking reflex, thereby passing flora to the baby.

An established way that mothers may pass on their healthy flora is via colostrum expressed prior to birth. Of course, not all pregnant women will be able to produce colostrum during pregnancy but, for those who can, lactation consultant Meg Stalnaker recommends hand expression while pregnant, storing the colostrum in the freezer, and bringing it to the hospital.

At the time of publication of this book, there has been research underway about the connection between the bacteria in the placenta and in the newborn.[15] Researchers at the Baylor College of Medicine found 300 different types of bacteria in the placenta that matched closely with the bacteria in the mouth, which is similar to the bacteria found in newborns' intestines. Further research may potentially reassure HBC mothers that their babies retain a fuller range of bacteria from their powerful placenta than previously thought.

Probiotics
Babies with poor gut health may be "colicky" or otherwise distressed, and it can be difficult for mothers to trust that their babies will be well and that

---

15   Science Translational Medicine 21 May 2014:Vol. 6, Issue 237, p. 237ra65
      http://stm.sciencemag.org/content/6/237/237ra65

they will successfully bond. A 2013 Netherlands research study indicated that newborns with colic tend to have less diverse and abundant mircrobiota than non-colicky babies.[16]

Many providers and mothers use probiotics in order to compensate for compromised flora (whether due to antibiotics, bathing, absence of vaginal secretions, and/or delayed breastfeeding). Carrie Thienes speaks to the positive effects of probiotics she has witnessed as an HBC mother and a nutritional therapist:

> Two major classes of bacteria populate our guts: residential and transient. A newborn ingests residential bacteria via passage through the vagina. Assuming the mother has a healthy gut biome (and is not receiving antibiotics during birth), these microbes begin to populate the baby's gut. Further population occurs from mother's milk, which also offers the beneficial, transient Lacto-based bacteria. Transient probiotic strains such as Lactobacillis and Acidophilous come through the diet and must be consistently ingested in order to keep the colonization active.

Thienes emphasizes that mothers should use live residential probiotics that are designed for their body type and have enteric coatings so that the probiotics get absorbed in the small intestine rather than being broken down in the stomach. These probiotics may also help soften the stool naturally and lessen bowel pain following major abdominal surgery. Thienes also suggests that a mother can re-innoculate her colon with probiotics by using an enema bag to rectally insert a quart of watered-down kefir, yogurt, or whey, and leaving in for 20 minutes. (See Appendix C, Resources for HBC Mothers and Families.)

My midwife encouraged me to give my baby probiotics in the hospital. I wouldn't have known otherwise. I did it covertly and it felt like one concrete thing I could do to help.
—Rachel (2009/HBC, Western U.S.)

---

16   Carolina de W. et al. *Pediatrics Official Journal of the American Academy of Pediatrics.* January, 2014. http://pediatrics.aappublications.org/content/early/2013/01/08/peds.2012-1449.abstract

Feed the baby first

Probiotics can improve the gut health of both the mother and baby, and babies whose mothers choose to and are able to breastfeed also reap the benefits of the microflora passed through breast milk. Most HBC mothers have knowledge of the benefits of breastfeeding and intend to breastfeed. However, the effects of a cesarean birth can impede these intentions and further interfere with mothers' experience of bonding.

Lactation consultant Cara Hafner offers a reassuring perspective for women facing severe breastfeeding challenges. "Breastfeeding is not all or nothing," she says. "Some breast milk is better than none. Women with low milk supply may use donor milk and/or a supplemental nursing system (SNS)." An SNS is a feeding device where a tube leads from a reservoir of milk or formula to the mother's nipple so that the mother and baby can experience the act of breastfeeding, even if the mother is not able to make milk.

When breastfeeding is not possible, donor milk may still be an option. Some hospitals offer pasteurized, screened donor milk for babies who need supplementation. For ongoing needs, milk from a milk bank may be an option as well as unpasteurized milk from a family member, friend, or other trusted source. "Breast milk from a trusted source contains bacteria that can help restore gut flora," says David Carroll, MD. "That's how humans did it for hundreds of thousands of years. There are risks, but these are low as long as the mother knows the source." (See Appendix C, Resources for HBC Mothers and Families for milksharing information.)

> Since 10 days old, she received over 22,000 ounces of donor milk at my breast from over 50 mothers of differently aged babies with a variety of diets. I say with absolute wonder that her digestive health has been amazing considering she received my IV antibiotics and she didn't go through the birth canal.
> —COURTNEY (2011/HBC, WESTERN U.S.)

With a severely low milk supply, I nearly gave up nursing. Ten days after birth, a hospital lactation consultant handed me a bottle and formula. Another consultant who understood my goals helped me use a supplemental nursing system. She said, "Every little bit of milk he gets from you matters. It's full of microflora that he needs." Even so, it didn't register with me until a year later that breast milk was giving him more than just calories and nutrition.
—Rachel (2009/HBC, Western U.S.)

A mother needs a way to feed her baby. When breastfeeding doesn't go well, isn't sustainable, or isn't possible, it is important to remember the larger context. "Feed the baby first," says lactation consultant Meg Stalnaker. "That's primary." When attempts to develop a breastfeeding relationship are overwhelming, it may deplete a woman's ability to mother her baby. For some, the most compassionate, healthy choice may be to not breastfeed. David Carroll recounts, "Everyone talks about how amazing breastfeeding is and how mothers have to do it for their babies. And it is amazing. But I see women who try their hardest yet are unable to breastfeed. These women feel so shameful, they're in tears in my office." There are numerous ways to nourish a baby. Some mothers use commercial formula, which may include probiotics; others make homemade formula. Carroll offers further reassurance: "You do what you can with what you're given to provide a healthy environment. I have patients who are born by cesarean, are unable to breastfeed, and need to have formula—and they turn out okay."

It cuts me to the core when mamas say negative things about formula or say, "At least I had breastfeeding." I felt so ashamed using formula that I would only take pumped milk to feed her in public. The idea of someone approaching me while I was in such a fragile state was enough to keep me home if I had no "real" milk to give her. I sometimes felt anxiety about not giving her all the benefits of breast milk, but I don't feel any change in connection with her.
—Leah (2012/HBC, Western U.S.)

Allow them to unwind themselves

For an HBC mother, facing the upfront issues of gut health and breastfeeding may challenge her experience of bonding with her child. Successfully navigating these issues may instill a deeper sense of confidence in herself and in her bond with her baby. As her baby grows, other challenges may present themselves, and each one may bring with it questions of her baby's wellness and bonding. Since many newborns express intense discomfort and pain as ways of communicating, it can be crucial for HBC mothers to use additional healing approaches.

Digestive issues may also arise from underlying physiological issues. Patty Wipfler, the founder and program director at Hand in Hand Parenting, has 40 years of experience helping parents and children form strong, emotionally connected relationships. She has seen many children with birth trauma "who turn out to be what people call colicky babies who don't settle well. Every time they eat there's intestinal pain or what seems like intestinal pain." A recent scientific perspective holds that the enteric nervous system (ENS) in the gut is the body's "second brain." The ENS, composed of an extensive network of neurons embedded in the gut tissue, controls digestion locally in the body, but it also sends signals to the brain, thereby affecting emotions and cognition. Regarding the "second brain," Wipfler notes that "tension in the body affects digestive ability. Children's digestive troubles affect how they feel about the world."

An interrupted birthing process—such as what occurs during an HBC— may result in some babies not feeling "complete" in their bodies. Passage through the vaginal canal prepares the baby's body to begin circulating blood through the heart and oxygen through the lungs. Donna Kellum-Patterson, LMT and retired doula, specializes in Three-fold Integrative Therapy (T-FIT), a practice that engages the body's self-corrective mechanisms to improve tissue mobility, bio-mechanics, and system balance, in the context of physical, soulful, and spiritual health. A baby born by cesarean, says Kellum-Patterson, may experience more of a "leap into the unknown" without any kind of biological transition. When Kellum-Patterson treats cesarean born babies, the release of tension in tissues throughout the body caused from this "leap" allows mothers and babies to better process the psychological and emotional imprint leading to overall wellness.

From the professionals we spoke with, the common thread is this: children need ways to somatically release trauma and to reset their systems and parents can support this healing.

Since many HBC mothers experience loss of control over what happens to their babies, it can be empowering for mothers to offer their own healing for their children. Carol Gray teaches mothers to do craniosacral therapy themselves:

> When mothers are holding their babies heart to heart, over the shoulder, babies will often arch their backs and lean away. A mother's first inclination might be to straighten the baby and hold him close so she doesn't drop him. I tell the mother that it's really good if her baby arches, because he knows how to get into certain positions to feel good. He is doing his cardinal movements and telling his birth story. One of the most helpful things we can do for these babies is to let them unwind themselves.

Patty Wipfler describes another unwinding practice which involves a relaxed, calm parent offering uninterrupted, mindful presence to a child for a defined period of time. The premise is that children, given full attention, will settle into a deep connection with their parent and find it safe to release hurts:

> Parents can share what I call "special time" when their child is alert and not hungry. A parent can receive whatever the baby communicates. The baby might show signs of discomfort, or might simply hold her parent's gaze for a long time. The parent doesn't try to find a cause for her actions. If special time is done shortly after a feeding, and the baby begins to cry while the parent is connecting with her, the parent can be fairly sure that if she cries, it's not about hunger— it's about the feelings she's carried into the present moment. Babies have to get rid of painful emotions so there's room for a more relaxed interpretation of reality. If a baby is working on fear, often her arms, legs, and chin will tremble; she'll cry loudly but there won't be tears. She'll begin to sweat and writhe; her body will contort and there will be tones of outrage. This is a common response to a rough birth. One hallmark of the feelings left by a traumatic experience is that no matter how many people were present and well intentioned at the time, the child feels that she experienced it alone. When infants re-experience these feelings, they need a relaxed, attentive adult to anchor them and say, "I'm with you."

HBC mothers have reported wonderful outcomes for their babies as a result of various forms of alternative body and energy work, from craniosacral therapy, to ritual re-birthing experiences, to holding deep presence for their children. Such approaches allow a baby to unwind while being lovingly supported. Mothers, partners, and birth professionals can all support babies in these ways.

> *Every bedtime from 6 to 9 months old, she would spend 15 minutes moving her head, turning on her belly, kicking. First I was annoyed because I really wanted her to go to sleep. When I realized she was doing the cardinal movements of birth, I was able to surround her with encouragement and tell her how happy I was that she was moving through her birth process. It only lasted a little longer after I was aware, and then her restlessness and urge were gone.*
> —Courtney (2011/HBC, Western U.S.)

> *It was amazing to watch her physically unfold during her craniosacral sessions. One time her face itself seemed to be changing. I told the practitioner, "She actually looks different now." She said, "In the birth canal their facial bones get molded. She didn't get that and she's getting that right now."*
> —Stephanie (2008, 2012/HBC; Northeastern U.S.)

> *Our baby was really struggling and we did biofeedback to understand what was going on. The results specifically pointed out birth related issues. He wasn't born in the way that he was expecting on a cellular level. Biofeedback, healing baths, baby-wearing, and lots of eye contact all helped him unwind.*
> —Erin (2009/HBC, 2012/HBAC; Western U.S.)

While this chapter highlights only a few healing approaches that HBC mothers have found helpful for their babies, there are many alternative healing modalities to choose from. It is important for families to find the approaches that work best and that support their babies to unwind, re-set, and feel connected and secure.

Baby meets scar: Shared storytelling

For newborns and infants, storytelling may begin by the mother telling the birth story, as with Mary Jackson's suggested approach earlier in this chapter. The baby may tell his own story by reenacting the cardinal movements of birth. Early on, there is a more distinct sense of storyteller and listener. As babies grow, storytelling becomes more collaborative. It may serve to heal, reframe, and strengthen the mother-child bond and empower them both.

When he was younger, we would look at the scar and tell a loving story about how he came out. But he said over and over how he wished he'd come out of my vagina. When our second son was born at home, he was there. Now he says he was born at home. I think it's healing for him so I am letting him own that for now.
—ERIN (2009/HBC, 2012, HBAC; WESTERN U.S.)

Each night when we were alone, I held her belly to belly, and visualized our cord, which oddly came from my vagina, connecting us. I matched my breathing with hers and imagined that breath coming from me into her and back to me. I silently repeated a mantra: "She came from my body, she grew in my belly, I nourish her, we are One." Eventually, the negative feelings decreased.
—BETHANIE (2009/HOSPITAL BIRTH, 2013/HBC; WESTERN U.S.)

She saw me putting oil on my scar and wanted to know where her scar was. I said, "This is my cesarean scar. I hope you never have one." Realizing how shameful that was, I said, "I'm sorry. You can have one if you want." Now when I put oil on my scar I say, "This is where you were lifted from my body. This is where you came out." I tell her how special and completely unexpected her birth was, with trickster, mischievous fox-like energy.
—COURTNEY (2011/HBC, WESTERN U.S.)

Let's play cesarean!
Babies instinctively play. As children grow, their play may take on new forms such as role-playing and verbal storytelling. Play can be the means through which children access their innate capacity to release old hurts and heal.

Midwife Mary Jackson works with children's birth stories through play therapy. Here she generalizes about the play she often sees:

Children have many common imprints, and there are challenges and gifts that come from every type of birth experience. The vaginally born toddler in a play tunnel often crawls directly out. The c-section born child crawls in the tunnel and may want to pop out the top or side, creating his own exit. The vaginally born toddler picks a toy and plays with it in the center of the room, and the c-section born toddler goes around the room's edges, checks for safety, and takes a toy to the center of the room. C-section born children have their antennas out to be alert and they often need preparation for transitions. They can figure out solutions quickly. Vaginally born children have to figure out the steps to find solutions, and babies born by cesarean can get right to the end result, because that is what happened to them.

Observing play can give insight into children's beliefs and experiences, and playing with them can help them rewrite their experiences. "Playlistening" is a practice similar to "special time" described by Patty Wipfler. Parents follow the child's lead and use play to help him release feelings and reconnect. The release and reconnection may come through laughter, tears, or a shift that isn't always immediately visible.

Donna Kellum-Patterson and her husband Bob Kellum-Patterson, a naturopathic physician, frequently work together with children and families who are recovering from traumatic birth experiences. They encourage parents to "trust their instincts and the ideas that come to them, even if they seem out of left field."

> One of her new favorite games is "playing cesarean." She gives her friends or herself cesareans or asks me to give her one. One time she said, "I'm having a baby, time to go to the hospital and I need you to cut it out." "Well," I said, "let's check and see where you are. Oh, you're at 10, I think you can push." She said, "If I could get it out, why would I be at the hospital?" Then I said, "I think you can do it. Why don't you just try pushing really hard and see what happens?" So she pretended to push and I lifted her newborn brother up between her legs. She was very excited.
> —Stephanie (2008, 2012/HBC; Northeastern U.S.)

> He'd try to crawl between the kitchen chair rungs, a space that was clearly big enough for him to fit through. But he'd get scared and gesture to me to pull him out and pick him up. I saw how much he wanted to get all the way through and realized that the rungs were like pelvic bones. It broke my heart each time I lifted him out. But I wanted to let him take his time, so I encouraged him and showed how his stuffed animals could go through. He initiated this play almost daily for several months until he eventually crawled all the way through himself. He looked so joyous and proud. Something completed for him because he never initiated this game again. It was healing for me that we

worked together and that I was able to be present in the way I wished I had been during his birth.
—Rachel (2009/HBC, Western U.S.)

My 4-year-old would bring me a pillow, baby doll, and blanket, and pretend I was pregnant and she was the midwife. Sometimes I pulled the doll out from the side or dropped it between my legs. Once after I had "birthed" a dozen babies, she wanted to be the baby. So she sat on my lap under the blanket and, when she was ready, I let her slowly drop to the floor. After a few times, she wanted to be born "the other way" so we did that a few times too, pulling her out sideways. She hasn't asked to play this game since.
—Misty (2008/HBC, 2011/HBAC; Western U.S.)

It's not about the dishes: Later childhood and beyond

Many HBC mothers express concern about getting off to a rough start with their babies and a rougher start finding support. Rose, mother of three, the oldest in his teens, offers a longer-term perspective on healing from potentially traumatic birth and babyhood experiences.

When I began to recognize how some of their behaviors are reflections of their birth experiences, it opened up a door to healing those experiences. For example, my second son, during labor, was in an awkward position that made birth impossible and, I imagine, was very uncomfortable for him. He was stuck, for at least eight hours, being forcibly pushed, with no exit. Now, when he is being stubborn and irrational, I let go of the present-day topic—dishes, home- work, his room— and, in my own heart, go back to his birth experience and acknowledge how difficult it is to feel like what is being asked of him is impossible. For a while, this process took a long time, often resulting with both of us holding each other, in tears, before the simple task that I had asked for was accomplished. But the tears were different than they had been before I began this practice. They were connecting tears. Over time, this "stuckness" of his has dissipated. It's been years since it's resurfaced.

The day after my first son's birth, the doctors couldn't find a vein to do a blood draw. My husband and I had to hold him down. He screamed until he went limp and essentially passed out. As a pre-teen, he again needed to have blood drawn. Before we went, I was thinking of him coming face to face with something that was part of his entrance into the world, which of course he didn't remember consciously. He was absolutely fine during the blood draw, but, in the privacy of our drive home, he asked me to stop the car. I pulled over with my emergency lights on. He stumbled out of the car and lay down in a fetal position in the grass. I held him and told him what happened when he was a baby. I explained that he didn't know then that the pain would end and didn't understand why the people who loved him the most had to hold him down. I told him that, now, as a young man, he could heal what happened in the past, because now he could meet it with understanding.

Taking those moments as they come, whether they're about dishes or blood draws or anything else, and speaking the truth in a way a child can understand, has been really powerful for our healing.

—Rose (2000, 2003/HBC, 2005/HBAC; Western U.S.)

Rose's description of supporting her children echoes several healing approaches discussed in this chapter: mindful listening, collaborative storytelling, and deep presence to help a child release trauma and reset his system. Above all, Rose's experiences illustrate how healing can occur throughout a person's lifetime.

Seeing our children clearly

While parents naturally want to help their children first, they must be well-resourced to be effective. Again and again, providers have stressed that when a mother receives support and experiences healing of any kind, her child ultimately benefits.

Parents also benefit from the type of supportive listening described throughout this chapter. In her work with families, Wipfler highlights:

> Parents need to tell the birth story, to protest, to fight, to be indignant and, with a listening partner, to cry and rage their way through the insults of the experience so they can see their child for who she is, and have a relationship free of stress rooted in the past. We need to help each other hold the perspective that although there are difficulties, we're alive. We made it. We get to have a good life with our children. Exchanging listening time with other parents helps us keep the big picture in focus.

Parents may gather support in numerous ways: talking with new and veteran parents, creating formal listening partnerships, counseling, new parent or specialized support groups, and making dedicated time for self-care and nourishing activities. Early on, small doses of any of these can go a long way towards helping to clear out hard feelings and can allow parents to be more available for their children.

> *I didn't go to support groups early on because I didn't want to take time away from my son, and I didn't want him to hear me talking negatively about his birth. Another HBC mom said point-blank, "He knows the whole story anyway. What if it's a good thing that he gets to see you as a strong mother getting support?" It took a long time for those words to sink in and for me to act on them.*
> —Rachel (2009/HBC, Western U.S.)

Trusting in the bond with a baby may take a while for some mothers, and that is okay. Beyond the birth itself, there are weeks and years to come, the entire primal period, a lifetime. When mothers get the support they need, they can more capably support their babies.

There are many ways to both acknowledge and transform a rough beginning. Regardless of the manner of birth, mothers can promote a healthy bacterial environment for themselves and their babies, choose best feeding options for their own situations, provide body work or other healing modalities, practice deep presence and supportive play to allow babies and children to tap into their own innate healing capacities, and use storytelling to manifest an empowered narrative for themselves and their children. Each moment offers the potential for healing and the celebration of wellness throughout our children's lives.

Chapter 10

Perinatal mood and anxiety disorders: The space between

After the birth, my room was the safest place in the world. But when I was overwhelmed by depression and anxiety, those four walls weren't safe enough. There were nights when I felt as though my body was coming apart, floating away, the space between every cell held shooting electricity. I felt raw, exposed, and, most of all, scared.

Entering motherhood in a whirlwind of pain, confusion, and abandonment hurt. At its worst, I felt like I was hanging on the lowest rung in a pit of despair, fighting desperately not to completely fall down. In order to raise my daughter, I had to let my body float away, feel that electricity, get overwhelmed by that fear. I had insomnia for five months because every evening was spent replaying my labor and surgery, trying to figure out how to dissipate unspent energy left behind when we stopped pushing and started cutting, and wondering why my midwife became distant and then disappeared.

There were a few times when I didn't want to be alive anymore. I didn't want to kill myself—that would take too much effort—I just wanted to be gone. To go to sleep forever. Anything but waking up to literal and figurative open wounds.

—Leah (2012/HBC, Western U.S.)

We most often hear the term *postpartum depression* when referring to women's mental health after childbirth. While this is the most common perinatal mood and anxiety disorder (PMAD), PMADs are a spectrum of disorders that can affect any woman during pregnancy or in the postpartum year. Mothers who have a difficult or traumatic birth, like an HBC, may be more likely to suffer from one or more PMADs and/or post-traumatic stress disorder (PTSD). Combine that risk with the normal lack of sleep that comes with a new baby, an inadequate support network that doesn't fully understand the needs of a mother grieving her birth experience, and the absence of self-care, and HBC mothers have a perfect mental health storm brewing.

Stigma about mental illness has always existed, and when mental and emotional disturbances happen to new mothers, quiet condemnation can prevent women from seeking the help they need. The shaming of mood and anxiety disorders can be subtle—birth professionals ignoring the possibility of PMADs and PTSD just as they may have ignored the possibility of homebirth cesarean. Or it can be blatant—mothers hearing they "just need to get over it and focus on the baby" from friends and family.

In this chapter, we show what PMAD screening by birth professionals can look like and why it is essential to holistic maternal care. We review symptoms and risk factors for all PMADs and postpartum PTSD, and we share stories from HBC mothers who have been through the mental health trenches. To gain more comprehensive information about PMADs and postpartum PTSD, refer to the books and reliable websites written by mental health professionals noted in the resource list in Appendix C.

Screening before and after birth

Birth professionals will only know if their clients are suffering from PMADs or PTSD if they are asking clients questions regardless of their mental health histories or birth outcomes. As care providers, it is impossible to observe most PMAD and PTSD symptoms during routine appointments—midwives can't perceive that a mother is obsessively washing her hands or that last night she was huddled in a corner of her bedroom wanting to cut her wrists. Since many mothers are reluctant to speak about their turbulent thoughts and emotions, the "don't ask and don't tell" cycle results in countless women not receiving support and treatment they desperately need.

> Without actually screening me, I was told by my midwife that I was "borderline and marginal." I wasn't somewhat anything—I was full on going crazy and no one was there to help me.
> —AMBER (2010/HBC, NORTHEASTERN U.S.)

Mental health screening is simple, and done by asking questions throughout a woman's care about her current, recent, and historical emotional health. On several occasions a midwife or doula should ask:

- How are you doing emotionally?

- How is your sleep? Are you able to sleep when the baby sleeps?

- How is your appetite?

- Do you have any questions for me about your emotions?

These inquiries are indicative of mental health because they provide the opportunity for women to begin to open up about their thoughts and emotions. This may allow mothers to start thinking about their emotions and actions from a perspective outside themselves. When asked these questions repeatedly during pregnancy and postpartum, women who started off reluctant to share their truths may become more comfortable answering honestly and thoroughly. Brooke Noli, a certified birth doula as well as a counselor who specializes in birth trauma, explains:

> During the perinatal year, women are about five times more likely to develop a mood and anxiety disorder than at any other time in their lives, so it just makes sense for midwives and doulas to screen for PMADs. If birth professionals don't screen, we inadvertently send the message that a woman's mental health is not as important as other aspects of her health. Screening gives birth professionals a chance to talk about how common PMADs are and to debunk some of the misinformation and stigma associated with them. Screening also gives us an opportunity to let suffering clients know that they are not alone, that there are effective treatments, and that help is available.

From responses to screening questions, birth professionals can prenatally develop a mental health baseline for each client and gain a sense of when to refer her to professionals and other local and national resources. When a woman screens positive for a PMAD or PTSD, the care provider's job is to validate her challenges, reassure her that what she is going through can be treated, and provide resources.

Treating PMADs is out of my scope of practice, so as a young midwife I never screened for them. It wasn't until I partnered with another midwife who prioritized screening that I realized how vital it is to women's care.
—DARIA SILVERMAN, CNM, NORTHEASTERN U.S.

In addition to feeling like identifying symptoms should be handled by a trained mental health worker, some birth professionals reported discomfort when mentioning PMADs and PTSD for fear that clients will feel singled out. Noli offers this observation:

> One of the main reasons birth professionals don't regularly screen is that we're afraid of frightening our clients or of planting seeds of negativity. Midwives and doulas deeply believe and trust in the natural birth process, and we view birth as a potential act of empowerment for women. Like cesarean birth, the thing about PMADs is that it doesn't easily fit with the natural birth model. Struggling with anxiety and depression is understandably not the image most people want to associate with pregnancy or the transition into motherhood, and midwives and doulas are no exception. We tend to invest in forwarding a mostly positive perception of the perinatal year because we think that's what will be most empowering to women, so discussions about difficult outcomes like cesarean or PMADs can sometimes fall by the wayside.

My records from my six-week postpartum appointment had a note that said I looked "well put together." My chart records from the appointment prior recorded that I told them I "wasn't right in my head." Yet I never received any information about PMADs.
—ANYA (2010/HBC, NORTHEASTERN U.S.)

When the conversation about PMADs, just like cesarean, is introduced during pregnancy and continued until the last postpartum appointment, women will understand that mental health screening is a routine part of childbirth education, holistic health, and the midwifery and doula models of care.

My midwife just wanted to make sure I wasn't going to hurt the baby. I would have liked her to be transparent about the screening, to tell me what she was screening me for and why. A more respectful way to screen for PMADs, rather

than trying to slip it into an already awkward conversation, would have been, "As you know, part of my job is to make sure that you have the support you need. So I'm going to ask you a series of questions that will help you and I determine if maybe you're experiencing more than just baby blues."
—DANA (2012/HBC, WESTERN U.S.)

If a woman perceives that her midwife or doula feels nervous or awkward when talking about PMADs, she is less likely to open up. In order to build comfort discussing and screening for PMADs, Noli offers this advice to birth professionals:

Develop a standard "script" that introduces the topic of PMADs and a list of assessment questions that fits well with their personal and professional style. Sometimes people look at an assessment tool like the Edinburgh Postnatal Depression Scale (EPDS) and think, "Jeez, this seems cold and clinical, and that's not the message I want to send to my clients." If an assessment tool is not a good fit for you, don't let that stop you from screening; just look for other options or create your own, because any assessment is better than none.

One midwife we spoke with said that when a mother seemed uncomfortable directly talking about her emerging PMAD symptoms, she would "ask her screening questions as the mother was changing her baby. This way I was sitting next to her, rather than directly across from her, and we were both focusing on her sweet baby while beginning the conversation about a serious issue." This seemingly offhanded approach can work well for women who are uncomfortable with the topic.

Years of working with women has granted me the wisdom to understand that mental health screening is essential. At every appointment I ask standard questions about her emotional state. If I feel there is something she isn't sharing, I ask more specific questions like, "Do you blame yourself for what happened during the birth? Do you ever feel panicky when you're with your baby?" Then I always, regardless of the answers, provide a list of therapists she can call. If I feel that a client is experiencing a PMAD, I give her that list and follow up to ensure she gets help.
—TARA JACKSON, BIRTH AND POSTPARTUM DOULA, NORTHEASTERN U.S.

In the weeks following birth, all women can be given a worksheet to fill out as part of their mental health screening. (See Appendix E, Screening Tools.) Midwives and doulas can tell the mother she will follow up with her at her next appointment and actually do so. If the mother is reluctant to complete the worksheet, the midwife or doula can make time during a regular appointment so she can focus on the PMAD assessment.

> *At our birth center we discuss a client's history of mood disorders prenatally and refer out to someone who deals specifically with those. For postpartum, we are working on having clients complete an Edinburgh Scale at least twice over the 6-8 weeks of care.*
> —Pamela Hines, retired midwife, Western U.S.

> *Before becoming a midwife, she was a mental health nurse and she was very concerned about me after my HBC. She scheduled longer appointments, told my husband what signs to look for and the difference between normal hormonal changes and postpartum depression. Having someone who actually cared about me and wasn't just filling in paperwork was amazing.*
> —Holly (2013/HBC, Australia)

> *Standard practice in our clinic is to educate families about all PMADs and inform them that onset may happen long after our care has ended. We provide resources, education, and screening regardless of birth outcome.*
> —Theresa Hyde, CNM, Canada

> *My husband called my midwives at six weeks postpartum because I was too embarrassed and proud to ask for help. They provided him with a suicide hotline and referred me to a postpartum depression support group. In that group I met strong, successful women who were blindsided by motherhood, women who were knocked on their butts by motherhood, and women who said very little about why they were there. These women had hard births, troubled relationships, breastfeeding issues, hormonal ebbs and flows. Being there made me feel a lot better about the fact that I was suffering.*
> —Emily (2011/HBC, Southern U.S.)

Birth professionals are not responsible for diagnosing or treating PMADs or PTSD. Their responsibility is to provide all women with resources, ask screening questions, and refer mothers to mental health professionals.

Treatment from professionals can include therapy and medication that is compatible with breastfeeding if the mother plans to continue nursing. Social support, validation, and alternative healing modalities such as acupuncture can augment her treatment plan as well. With proper care, all PMADs can be cured, but if left untreated, they can last years.

> There must be better awareness and more tolerance of using pharmaceuticals and professional therapy to help mothers. Too often the midwifery approach is to only discuss supplements or alternative therapies without referral to someone skilled in the mental health field. Many times alternative therapies cannot touch what women are dealing with and it's our responsibility to refer out to mental health professionals.
> —PAMELA HINES, RETIRED MIDWIFE, WESTERN U.S.

Why women don't disclose

Despite the best educational efforts from the birth team, often HBC mothers are still in shock, grief, and trauma in the early weeks after birth, and most likely can't differentiate normal mood changes from PMADs or PTSD. They may also hear that they have a healthy baby and that is the most important thing, or they may fear that their baby will be taken away from them if they do admit to feeling unstable. This leads to mothers hiding their symptoms, desperately trying to "hold it together" and "move on."

> I couldn't eat or shower and my partner didn't know what to do with me. But when it came time for my midwifery appointments, I cleaned myself up and slapped on a smile. They had no idea I was so bad.
> —SABINA (2010/HBC, 2012/HB; NORTHEASTERN U.S.)

> During pregnancy, my midwives provided a written questionnaire about my mental health. I failed to mention my father's severe anxiety, paranoid behavior, and his bi-polar, manic-depressive issues. I didn't talk about my sister's bipolar disorder or my own depression and brush with attempted suicide as a teenager.
>
> My midwives only saw a happy and positive client. But I had real and deep worry about my baby being taken away, along with forgetting I had a baby, and fear about my husband dying. I only told them verbally that I was worried about my postpartum, but I didn't actually provide them with any real evidence to back it up. I was also prideful about my abilities to handle what

might happen. Plus, my mother-in-law came with my husband and me to my
appointments, so I wasn't going to admit my fears or history in front of her.
—EMILY (2007/HBC, SOUTHERN U.S.)

When birth professionals are able to offer a solo visit to clients in the second trimester, this may allow mothers to feel more at ease discussing their mental health history and current emotional state. Wendy Davis, psychotherapist and the executive director of Postpartum Support International, offers that:

> There is so much benefit to moms or partners asking for help and doing so as early as possible. The earlier they reach out, the easier it is to intervene and prevent escalation. Families can connect with reliable support and resources, allowing them to talk with informed providers to prevent misinformation and unnecessary shame and fear. With solid information, encouragement, and treatment, mothers are able to find relief and increase positive experiences for themselves and their children.

Types of perinatal mood and anxiety disorders

The following are descriptions of the risk factors and symptoms of perinatal mood and anxiety disorders. Symptoms for all PMADs except psychosis can begin at any time during pregnancy or the first year postpartum.

It is important to note that most postpartum women have many of these PMAD symptoms at one time or another. Normal hormonal changes combined with a homebirth cesarean create disturbances in emotions and thoughts. It is when a woman experiences multiple symptoms almost every day over the course of several weeks that a PMAD may be present.

The risk factors and symptoms of each PMAD are not listed in a particular order.

Baby blues, while extremely common, is not included in this section because it does not require treatment. The symptoms of baby blues may include feeling disappointed, crying for no apparent reason, and irritability. These feelings are mild and end quickly, usually by the first two weeks following birth.

POSTPARTUM DEPRESSION (PPD)

Postpartum depression felt like I was doing everything wrong. I had no faith in my ability to parent or be a wife. I didn't know how to interact with my family, friends, or even strangers. I couldn't sleep at night because I felt like if I did, something terrible would happen to my son. Yet I would look at him and feel no connection, only intense fear. Every day I thought I should just leave, that my husband and baby would both be better off without me.
—LIBBY (2011/HBC, 2013/VBAC TRANSPORT; MIDWESTERN U.S.)

Depression in the postpartum year is the most common PMAD, with research showing an estimated prevalence rate of 14%, though we can assume that many cases of Postpartum Depression (PPD) go undiagnosed every year.[17]

It is impossible to accurately forecast which women will have PPD and which will come out of a birth feeling emotionally stable, but these factors can put women at a higher risk for developing PPD:

- Personal or family history of clinical depression and/or anxiety disorders

- Inadequate social support including relationship and financial stresses

- Complications in fertility, miscarriage, pregnancy, birth, feeding of the baby, and/or the health of the baby

- Current thyroid imbalance

- Sensitivity to hormonal changes around puberty and/or birth control

Symptoms are different for every woman, but may include:

- Apathy toward the baby

---

17   (1) Katherine L. Wisner, MD, MS, etal, *Onset Timing, Thoughts of Self-harm, and Diagnoses in Postpartum Women With Screen-Positive Depression Findings* http://archpsyc.jamanetwork.com/article.aspx?articleid=1666651)

- Inability to sleep when given the opportunity or disturbed sleep patterns

- Loss of appetite or overeating

- Intense feelings of overwhelm, despair, anger, guilt, and/or shame

- Volatile emotions

- Detachment and depersonalization

- Inability to concentrate

- Irritability and anger

- Thoughts of self-harm

Elise wished she could have birthed her baby in her bedroom, not in the operating room. When her midwife asked how she felt about her HBC, Elise talked about her shame and guilt and how she felt like she let everyone down. She never mentioned depression or even feeling sad. Elise's midwife was familiar with PPD, having experienced it herself with all three of her children, and she referred Elise to a social worker who specialized in perinatal mental health. Elise seemed interested in the referral during her appointments but never called the social worker. At every visit her midwife normalized her PPD symptoms and discussed the relief Elise would feel if she decided to seek help. Because of her midwife's persistence, Elise finally scheduled an appointment and began regular bi-weekly counseling sessions.

Postpartum depression or anxiety may spiral into thoughts of self-harm and suicide, and do require clinical support from a trained mental health professional. It is never enough, for example, to recommend that a depressed or anxious mother take Vitamin D supplements or begin an exercise routine. In addition to local and national mental health resources given prenatally and re-introduced postpartum, birth professionals must refer clients to qualified professionals who specialize in pregnancy and postpartum mental health.

POSTPARTUM ANXIETY AND POSTPARTUM PANIC DISORDER

I was intensely paranoid that someone was going to take my baby while we were jogging. I was constantly looking over my shoulder, thinking she would be snatched away from me, to the point that I was really thinking about the route I would take and the amount of people around. I definitely had invasive thoughts.
—SKY (2008/HBC, NORTHEASTERN U.S.)

A large public health research study found that up to 66% of the women who screened positive for depression had concurrent anxiety or panic.[18] Anxiety or panic may be experienced alone or in addition to depression, and risk factors include personal or family history of anxiety or panic, previous trauma, or a current thyroid imbalance.

The symptoms for generalized postpartum anxiety may include:

- Constant worry or feeling that something bad will happen

- Fears of going crazy and/or being alone

- Racing thoughts

- Disturbances of sleep and appetite

- Continuous need to do something

Postpartum panic disorder, a subset of anxiety, also includes recurring panic attacks along with the above symptoms.

Peter casually mentioned that earlier in the week Aubrey cleaned the house, cooked dinner, and bathed the dogs, all while caring for their new baby. Aubrey's midwife asked her how she was feeling during all that activity and what she was thinking as she was completing those tasks. Aubrey shared that her mind is sometimes unable to rest and she feels like she needs to

18   (2) Katherine L. Wisner, MD, MS, etal, *Onset Timing, Thoughts of Self-harm, and Diagnoses in Postpartum Women With Screen-Positive Depression* Findings http://archpsyc.jamanet-work.com/article.aspx?articleid=1666651)

constantly be doing something. When she sits alone with her baby, she can only think about the operating room. She said that her mind kept returning to thoughts and fears of the future, even when she tried to focus on something else. Her midwife assured the new family that Aubrey's feelings are common after a difficult transport and birth. She encouraged Aubrey to seek professional help and followed up at every appointment to see how therapy was working for her.

POSTPARTUM OBSESSIVE-COMPULSIVE DISORDER (OCD)

I went OCD and secretly stuck a scale in my closet, weighing my son every hour. My best friend noticed I wasn't right and told my husband.
—ELLIE (2006/HBC, 2010/HBAC; WESTERN U.S.)

Postpartum obsessive compulsive disorder (OCD) is another subset of anxiety and is more common than once thought, with an estimated prevalence rate of 5% of new mothers.[19] The risk factor is a personal or family history of OCD.

As indicated by its name, obsessions (persistent thoughts or images) and compulsions (actions to reduce the obsessions) are both present with OCD.

Symptoms may include:

- Intrusive, repetitive thoughts or images (obsessions)

- Repetitive actions, usually attempts to avoid the fear (compulsions)

- An understanding that the intrusive thoughts and actions are odd and don't make sense

- A sense of horror about the thoughts, fears, or images

---

19   (3) Brandes et al. (2004) *Postpartum Onset Obsessive-Compulsive Disorder: Diagnosis & Management. Archives of Women's Mental Health*, vol. 7; is. 2: 99-102. http://link.springer.com/article/10.1007/s00737-003-0035-3)

- Fear of being alone with the baby

- Hyper vigilance about protecting the baby

Laura was fixated on her baby's gut flora and she asked the same questions about cesarean and IV antibiotics at every midwifery appointment. Over the course of a few weeks, Laura's questions become more frequent and the midwives began receiving frantic calls about probiotics and the baby's digestion, and how her HBC might impact her baby's long-term health. Her midwives suspected she was suffering from postpartum OCD and put together a resource document specifically addressing this PMAD. By providing gentle encouragement, Laura was able to seek help from a therapist who, in addition to weekly appointments and medication that was compatible with breastfeeding, also enrolled Laura in an outpatient support group.

BIPOLAR DISORDERS: MANIA, BIPOLAR DEPRESSION, AND MANIC DEPRESSION

> I would swing between the charismatic social event planner in my new moms' group to such deep depression and lethargy that I couldn't attend the next day's playgroup I had organized. I felt completely manic and out of control.
> —SELMA (2009/HBC, SOUTHERN U.S.)

The postpartum period is a high-risk time for recurrence of previous bipolar symptoms, while research shows that anywhere from 10-26% of postpartum women develop first-time symptoms on the spectrum of bipolar depression.[20] Risk factors are a personal or family history of bipolar disorders.

In addition to depression, symptoms may include:

- Mild to extreme mania

- Mixed moods, from despair to elation

- Highly irritable

---

20   (4) Viguera A, et al. *Risk of Recurrence in Women with Bipolar Disorder During Pregnancy,* Am J Psychiatry 2007, (164)12

- Increased talkativeness

- Risky and/or impulsive behavior

- Racing thoughts

- Disrupted sleep patterns and decreased need for sleep

In the weeks following birth, Chary reported feeling euphoric and ecstatic. Her birth team was surprised by her happiness since they knew how much Chary wanted to have her baby at the birth center. As they spent more time with her, they realized that her joy seemed a little different than the happiness most new mothers usually feel—there was a wild and pressured component to it. Her midwives set aside time at every appointment to ask questions about her sleep patterns, thoughts, and plans for the future. Her birth team was able to reconnect Chary with the therapist she'd seen before she was pregnant, and she was able to begin treatment that included medication and weekly therapy sessions.

POSTPARTUM PSYCHOSIS

> *My chest itched, I couldn't sleep, and I made plans to hide my baby from the world.*
> —ALECIA (2009/HBC, UNITED KINGDOM)

Psychosis is more rare than depression or anxiety and extremely serious, occurring after 1 to 2 per thousand births.[21] The onset of symptoms is sudden, usually within the first two to four weeks after birth, and it requires emergency medical treatment. Wendy Davis says that:

> Women with psychosis might at first appear depressed or anxious, or perhaps have a confusing heightened energy and bursts of ideas. They may fluctuate from this manic state to extreme and troubling disruption in their thinking and perceptions. The biggest difference between psychosis and anxiety is that anxious women are very frightened of their

---

21   (5) Beck, CT. (2001) *Predictors of Postpartum Depression: An Update.* Nursing Research, 50(5): 275-285

thoughts and images, while a woman in a psychotic state might even appear calm. An anxious mom may be afraid that she'll hurt her baby, while a psychotic mom might think, for example, that bringing her baby to heaven is the very best thing to do. To the woman in a psychotic state, the elaborate thoughts make sense to her, even if they are horrifying or dangerous to others.

A personal or family history of a bipolar disorder or a previous psychotic episode are risk factors for psychosis.

Symptoms may include:

- Delusions

- Hallucinations

- Paranoia

- Confusion

- Hyperactivity

- Rapid mood swings

- Suicidal or other intrusive thoughts about harming the baby and/or family that seem like a good idea and make sense to the woman

Abigail's midwives said they were concerned that she had postpartum depression and recommended that Abigail begin therapy. Abigail's partner, Theresa, hired a postpartum doula to help care for the new baby. Theresa also secretly hoped that the doula would keep Abigail from feeling so lonely and anxious. The doula grew concerned after Abigail frequently reported that it felt like bugs were crawling over her incision and she kept forgetting to eat. She was sometimes frightened and was staying up late spending hours on the Internet researching cesareans. Once she said there were "clues in there." One morning Theresa found her in the kitchen stretched on the floor in a yoga pose with the baby next to her. She had been there all night. Abigail seemed caught in a dream and gave a rambling answer about her purpose when Theresa asked what she was doing. Later she accused Theresa and the doula of keeping secrets and planning to take the baby from her.

After one shift when Abigail suddenly stopped talking to her, the doula phoned Theresa from her car, explained that she felt Abigail needed urgent help, and asked her to come home immediately. Theresa and the doula were able to convince Abigail that they needed to go to the emergency room together, telling her that they were worried about her fears and her lack of sleep. They were so relieved that she agreed to go, although she was suspicious and reluctant and it took constant convincing. While they waited there, Abigail became agitated and cried, seeing and feeling the bugs again. As she whimpered and hit the imagined bugs away, the doctor explained to Abigail that they wanted to admit her to help her sleep and stop the feeling of bugs. A nurse told them that she might be having all these scary symptoms from the sleep deprivation and exhaustion. Abigail didn't want to stay at first and looked scared, but she was so exhausted that she allowed them to hospitalize her for treatment.

SELF-HARM AND SUICIDAL IDEATION

> When I told my therapist my plan to go away, that my son would be fine without me, she told me he would never be okay—that he would spend the rest of his life not being okay, needing me. There was something about the way she said it that shocked me back to life and I realized suicide was a bad idea.
> —ANN (2011/HBC, MIDWESTERN U.S.)

Self-harm and suicidal ideation are not an actual PMAD by themselves, however thoughts of self-harm, a preoccupation with thoughts of suicide, planning a suicide, and/or attempting suicide can be symptoms of various PMADs. In a 2012 study of 10,000 postpartum depressed women, a startling 20% had thoughts of self-harm or suicide.[22] Signs that a woman is at an increased risk of suicide may include:

---

22   (5) Katherine L. Wisner, MD, MS, et al, *Onset Timing, Thoughts of Self-harm, and Diagnoses in Postpartum Women With Screen-Positive Depression Findings* http://archpsyc.jamanetwork.com/article.aspx?articleid=1666651

- Talking about feeling hopeless, trapped, in unbearable pain, being a burden, wanting to die, or that the baby would be better off without her

- Self-imposed isolation

- Extreme mood swings

- Impulsivity

- The means and specific plans to commit suicide

The times that Jessica and her husband fought were the worst. Jessica could handle the depression and anxiety after the birth, but when she and Fred would argue she felt so alone, like her world was pulled away from her. She could only think about holding a knife to her wrists and felt that the connection between her incision and the knife in her hand was poetic. Since she failed at even going into labor and was unable to make enough milk to feed her baby, she felt like she didn't deserve to be a mother. She was so afraid her baby would be taken away if she also failed at killing herself—just like her baby was taken away after the surgery. She didn't know what to do or whom to talk to. It was Fred who knew Jessica wasn't okay and sat with her as she called therapists from the list their doula gave them. It was Fred who drove her to her weekly appointments and it was Jessica who, with therapy, medication, and much needed permission and support to discontinue breastfeeding, gained a new perspective about her HBC and becoming a mother.

POSTPARTUM POST-TRAUMATIC STRESS DISORDER (PTSD)

I was so on edge for months after the birth that I would jump at the slightest sounds. I had to sleep on a towel to soak up my sweat from reoccurring nightmares about the ambulance ride to the hospital. And my PTSD was always triggered during doctor appointments.
—DEVYN (2007/HBC, 2013/HB; WESTERN U.S.)

Postpartum PTSD is not considered a PMAD, but women may experience PTSD along with other mood and anxiety disorders. A trauma during childbirth, like a cesarean or a perceived or real near-death experience, and a trauma history are risk factors for PTSD. An estimated 1-6% of women experience PTSD following childbirth.[23]

PTSD symptoms may include:

- Intrusion: Frequent re-experiencing of the traumatic event(s) through flashbacks or nightmares

- Avoidance: Evading stimuli of the traumatic event(s) such as visual and olfactory reminders and/or people or locations associated with the HBC

- Increased arousal: Disrupted sleep patterns, hypervigilance, and/or an exaggerated startle response

- Anxiety and panic attacks

Penny is a midwife who provides attentive and caring postpartum support, especially to mothers who were not able to birth at home. Because she felt her care was so nurturing and thorough, it was difficult for her to make the correlation between her client's births and the possibility that they might suffer from PTSD. After one of Penny's clients had a homebirth cesarean that left the mother reeling from postpartum depression and PTSD, Penny began educating herself and her apprentices about the different PMADs and postpartum PTSD. She started to understand that her care could not prevent her clients from experiencing their births as traumatic. Instead of equating good midwifery care with positive mental health outcomes, she added into the equation the mother's perception of her birth and her history of life experiences prior to childbirth.

Partners support the mother

Partners are learning to parent a new baby too. They are feeling overwhelmed by the responsibilities and sleep disturbances of caring for the newborn. They may feel isolated as they cope with the birth, and may not understand or have the resources to support the complexity of the mother's mental health.

---

23   (3) Beck C. 2004. *Post-traumatic stress disorder due to childbirth: the aftermath.* Nursing Research 53(4): 216-24

I was exhausted, isolated, confused, and depressed. But I couldn't take care of those things because I had to support my wife who was far worse than me.
—Moe, partner of Ezra (2008/HBC, Western U.S.)

Sometimes I took her depression personally, like she blamed me for her pain. It was hard to deal with her, our baby, and my own anxiety about being a new dad.
—Travis, partner of Lan (2010/HBC, Western U.S.)

He felt isolated, disappointed, and scared. Six months after the birth, before he'd come home from work, he'd stop at a bar to shore himself up, to deal with me and this kid. I wanted to pass off the baby the minute his hand reached the doorknob, but instead we would argue about who had suffered more that day.
—Kim (2001/HBC, Midwestern U.S.)

While partners care for themselves, they must also care for the HBC mother. Counselor Brooke Noli believes that most women with a PMAD need:

> understanding, reassurance, and patience from their partners. The only way that partners can offer those things is if they are well informed about their loved one's condition. There is still a lot of misinformation and stigmatization out there, and if partners fall prey to these common myths, it can just add to an already difficult situation.

> Women need their partners to reassure them that the condition is nobody's fault and that they are not to blame. They need partners to tell them again and again they are good mothers and that things *will* get better. They need help with childcare, household chores, and with getting sufficient amounts of sleep. They need partners who are willing to listen, who are patient with the process of healing, and who don't feel constantly driven to try to "fix it." And they need partners who support their efforts to get help from therapists, support groups, and medical providers.

In addition to their role as caretakers, partners may also be suffering from postpartum mood and anxiety disorders themselves. Birth professionals can help normalize a mentally turbulent experience for partners by educating them that postpartum mood and anxiety disorders are also common for partners. As partners learn their own personal balance of self-care while supporting the new mother, they can access local and national resources designed specifically for partners. (See Appendix C, Resources for HBC Mothers and Families.)

Voices from the space between

I was vicious, I wasn't myself. All I could do was hysterically cry, and I couldn't function, I couldn't even drive. I felt a complete existential crisis—I didn't believe in homebirth, midwifery, cesarean, or God. I felt like I lost everything.
—ELLIE (2006/HBC, 2010/HBAC; WESTERN U.S.)

I spiraled into a postpartum depression so deep, I thought I might never get out. I felt like a complete failure. I hated myself, I hated my body. I realized I had been hallucinating, but I had no idea for how long. I also had the shakes, jitters, ticks, and I was nauseous and dizzy.

My depression and anxiety stemmed from the homebirth cesarean. My body felt like it had been taken over, used, damaged, and put back together wrong. So I was scared of healing wrong. I was scared of not healing at all. My world had been a snow globe shaken around and I was left to deal with it. I did not know how to be a mother, and my very first act in motherhood ended terribly out of control.
—CAROL (2012/HBC, WESTERN U.S.)

I'd be sitting in bed breastfeeding my daughter and my mouth would go dry, my ears would ring, and my heart would beat so fast, I thought I would die. My palms would get so sweaty that I could barely hold my baby and I'd get so cold I'd start to shake. Before I understood that I was having a panic attack, I thought it was a heart attack.
—LYDIA (2008/HBC, SOUTHERN U.S.)

It was impossible to leave the house—the anxiety was so real. I would forget to bring basic items on short errands and end up having a panic attack and coming right home, shaken and upset for hours. On the front and back doors I hung a list of things to do before leaving. They were small things I learned in my support group that would help me feel more confident, like brushing my teeth or wearing earrings. Once I realized I didn't need the list anymore, that I could leave the house and be prepared without reading it line by line, I took it down.

At the very worst of times, I found the reason to keep going and pull through because of my little guy. He needed me more than anyone ever has. While that thought spurred many anxious thoughts and fearful realities, it also grew within me a drive I did not have before.
—EMILY (2007/HBC, SOUTHERN U.S.)

The care mothers need

If left untreated, PMADs and PTSD can have serious and long-term consequences for mothers that will affect the overall health and stability of a family. Thankfully, PMADs and PTSD are highly responsive when properly treated by mental health professionals. Birth professionals need to ask thoughtful questions about a mother's emotional health throughout care and refer her to local and national resources, helping her to seek the support she deserves.

Birth Professionals' Quick Guide to PMADs and Postpartum PTSD

- Self-educate about the risk factors and symptoms of all PMADs and PTSD.

- Screen all mothers, regardless of mental health history, appearance, and birth outcome.

- Provide local and national mental health resources during pregnancy and again after birth.

- During a client's solo visit, inquire about her past and current mental health.

- Refer clients, including partners, to mental health professionals.

- Follow up with clients to ensure they are getting help that works for them.

- Provide screening worksheets and make time for mothers to complete them.

Chapter 11

In the end, it's everyone finding themselves

How do you heal from your experience of being wounded by life and move forward with your heart open? How do you reach out in kindness and love to others and yourself? How do you keep doing that if you've been traumatized? The most inspiring answer is that we learn to forgive. But before we are able to forgive, we must acknowledge that something painful occurred. Then we can identify our unenforceable rules around that experience.

It's fine to work hard, wish, and hope for a homebirth, but if you demand a homebirth and make that an unenforceable rule, you set yourself up to be hurt, disappointed, and angry. If you have unenforceable rules about how birth is supposed to be, then challenge them. With that challenge comes the act of digging down and taking responsibility to find a way to be healthy and at ease in your life in the face of a homebirth cesarean.

—JENNIFER GADDY, NATUROPATHIC DOCTOR AND INSTRUCTOR OF BIO/PSYCHO/SPIRITU-AL INTEGRATION, WESTERN U.S.

As the first HBC anniversary draws close, birth stories are rehashed and often painful memories resurface. Women's relationships with their cesarean scars breathe life into the struggles they may have thought they healed from. HBC women's own roles within the natural birth community can become more emotionally complicated as they seek new ways to define their out-of-hospital birth that ended in surgery. In this chapter, we explore healing in the years following a homebirth cesarean.

Greater awareness of the journey

A woman's feelings about her HBC evolve as she continues to integrate her birth and grow as a mother. Some women struggle to make sense of their journey, others arrive at a place of great understanding, and some focus on specific aspects of healing, like forgiveness. No matter the route, hopefully mothers are able to do their best to make sense of their difficult sojourn.

Having a homebirth cesarean was one of the best things to ever happen to me. In the end it was a profound healing for my arrogance around natural birth and homebirth; it really woke me up. It took me eight years to recover, to come to a place of complete peace and understanding about what it meant to me to have a cesarean after planning a homebirth. Not everyone has to take that kind of journey, but for some reason I did. It took a long time to heal and come "home" to myself because the psychic shattering was so great.
—Pam England (1982/HBC, 1990/HBAC, Birthing from Within author and founder; Western U.S.)

I didn't choose well with my midwife. I didn't choose the right people to care for my son or for me. I'm in the process of forgiving myself for these things.
—Sage (2008/HBC, Western U.S.)

I don't believe other HBC moms are failures, but I still feel that I am. I'm guessing this is a common thread through us all—the sympathy for one another and the inability to let go of our own guilt. This is my continuing emotional battle, and I hope to someday have the capacity to forgive myself.
—Alexis (2011/HBC, Midwestern U.S.)

I'm trying to be more comfortable telling people I hated my birth and that's okay because I love my daughter. It wasn't awesome. It wasn't magical. It wasn't all these things I had expectations about. I've gotten okay paying homage to that.
—Alissa (2011/HBC, Western U.S.)

I was angry, depressed, and lonely about my HBC but now, years later, I don't feel so wounded by the experience. I'm continually working on turning it around and finding the humor, the empowering moments, the lessons learned. I have explored what my expectations were, looked at the big picture, and saw what I wanted to hold onto. I've gotten to know my body better, and I am still strengthening it. I can talk more objectively about my HBC without a wave of emotions coming over me every time. I don't feel so disempowered by my birth, or like if I talk about it that I'm betraying the homebirth world.
—Erin (2007/HBC, 2009/CS after attempted VBAC, 2011/RCS; Western U.S.)

I put myself completely in the hands of my midwife. I believed everything she said. Then, when things went "wrong," I felt betrayed. I've learned that we are all responsible for our own births. We are not in control and neither are our midwives. We're all just humans responding with the tools we have in the moment.
—BETH (2009/HBC, WESTERN U.S.)

The scar that marks us

HBC women have physical scars to show for their birthing efforts—some vertical, most horizontal, occasionally keloided, others bumpy or invisible. A woman's focus on her scar changes with time and she may feel increased shame and sadness as she realizes it's not vanishing the way she had hoped. Or she may continue to ignore touching the evidence of her surgery, while another mother might be able to find peace with the scar that marks her.

I used to hate my scar because I felt gutted like a prey animal. I hated looking at it and how my stomach hung over it. I compulsively touched it because it was so large and different and I did my best not to think about it. But I've now found some peace with it. I've learned more about myself since the shock of my cesarean and that has helped me accept the scar, even if I will never like it.
—HEATHER (2009/HBC, MIDWESTERN U.S.)

Since my scar is a long vertical one that extends to within an inch of my navel, I see it each day as I dress and accept it as I do any other of my less desirable physical attributes.
—PIPER (1982/HB, 1987/HBC; MEXICO)

I didn't want to acknowledge it for a long time. It was a symbol of a very sad time for me. Now, I view it as a sign of my selflessness and strength.
—CHRISTINE (2009, 2012/HBC; NORTHEASTERN U.S.)

My scar blends into the scenery like a crack in the wall of a familiar room. I don't remember what it was like not to have it. I touch it lovingly and with special care. My son loves my scar. It's like a memorial to his existence—proof that we are connected.
—BETH (2009/HBC, WESTERN U.S.)

My scar was the first mark left on my body. I felt as though I had been pristine and whole before the cesarean and then after I felt marked and less of a woman. It was a daily reminder that I was not quite good enough. It faded over time and when I was pregnant again it was nearly invisible. After my second HBC it healed differently, lumpy, and with an uneven texture. It hasn't faded yet and it now has a little overhang. Maybe in time I will learn to love it, but right now, it is a leering reminder of my lost homebirths.
—Bronwyn (2008, 2011/HBC; South Africa)

I don't touch it. I don't look at it. I avoid feeling or thinking about it.
—Rebecca (2012/HBC, Southern U.S.)

I'm not squeamish, and I love the ways of my body, so my incision site was never a source of direct trauma. I find power in my scar. It's where I feel my womb energy leaving my body and flowing towards my daughter. I'm grateful that this is the way I'm able to speak of it.
—Sue (2010/HBC, Western U.S.)

After my first HBC, I hated my scar because it felt like it didn't belong there. I wasn't supposed to be one of the people who needed a c-section. After my second HBC, I felt like a failure and my scar was a constant reminder of that. Since my third HBC, I've been embarrassed about my lower stomach area. It's not so much the scar, but the flap of skin that overhangs it. I never used to mind being naked but now, thanks to my cesareans, I no longer feel beautiful. I find myself putting my hand over my lower stomach when my husband sees me at intimate times. It's the only part of my body that I would be tempted to change if I could.
—Laura (2003, 2008, 2011/HBC; Midwestern U.S.)

In the beginning, I disassociated from my scar and talked about and treated it like it was separate from me. I decided to do the whole "fake it 'til you make it" thing and massaged it while practicing deep breathing and relaxation. After a while I went from angry to neutral to loving it.
—Leah (2012/HBC, Western U.S.)

My son is in the tub, curious for the first time about his belly button. By the look on his face, I can see that he finds the story of the umbilical cord as fantastical as any fairy tale written to initiate children into the impossible.

He asks a question that makes it clear he has heard about cesarean birth, something we have never discussed. I lower the elastic of my underwear and show him the small, raised smile of a scar.

This is where you came through mommy into the world, I tell him. The doctors helped cut me right here so you could be born.

I reassure myself: this can't be any more gruesome or confusing for a 3-year-old to hear than what happens in vaginal birth.

He asks if I have a belly button that once tied me to my mommy. He wants to know if every person has a belly button. He is trying to make sense of how our bodies connect and release us.

Until now, I had held my indelible cesarean evidence in loneliness and shame—a secret sign that I had failed at my most important job.

Suddenly, it occurs to me that a belly button is a scar that everyone has. I am not alone in the grief or the brutality of being human. We are all required to let go of the people we love sooner or later. Every one of us is marked by this crossing.
—Written by Sage (2008/HBC, Western U.S.)

The stories we tell, the healing we offer

HBC mothers have a difficult time comprehending why and how their births traversed so far from their plans. "Why it happened is sometimes understandable in retrospect, but not necessarily in the moment," says Donna Patterson-Kellum, LMT. Because of this, the stories women share about their births reflect their perception of the experience in the moment of telling, the narrative continually evolving over time. Every HBC woman's grief is unique in its causes, trajectory, and length, but some commonalities do exist.

Midwife and doula Barbara Herrera lists on her Navelgazing Midwife blog birth mourning stages she discovered in attending births for women who experience unexpected outcomes.[24] She labels these stages beginning with

---

24   Herrera, B. E. (2008, February 11). *The Gray, Grey Messenger: Recovery.* Message posted to http://navelgazingmidwife.squarespace.com/navelgazing-midwife-blog/2008/2/11/the-gray-grey-messenger-recovery.html

adoration and ending with assimilation and preparation. Along the way are disbelief, sadness for naiveté, anger and blame, sadness for the experience, reframing, and acceptance.

It can be helpful to think of these stages as a framework for the grieving, not a "one size fits all" approach to progressing through the mourning process. Over time, a mother will gain some distance from her birth, and the perspective that the distance yields allows her to reframe her experience. In her blog Herrera describes reframing this way:

> When women can take all of the information they've learned and superimpose it over the birth experience, they have begun to reframe. To be able to see the situation from different angles, from different points of view, even from her different lifetimes, all of these help a woman to adjust her thoughts about how and why her birth happened the way it did. I see reframing as an enormous leap towards healing. Reframing doesn't minimize, erase, or invalidate the pain and trauma a woman might have experienced. Instead, it softens the colors, blunts the swords, and begins to put things in the greater context of her life.

When a mother has begun to contextualize her birth experience, she may use that newfound point of view to promote her wisdom and shape a new, more triumphant story. She may find that in telling her story to others, instead of anger, blame, or disbelief being the underlying emotion, she describes her birth in terms of having done her best and having the ability to look with love and compassion at the scars left behind. The mother may eventually move into the last phase of birth mourning, which is assimilation and preparation. Herrera describes this stage as pulling the birth into her heart: "She embraces it for all the lessons, the beauty that it was. She finds immense pride in her strength and feels crone-like, having seen 'death,' but still pressing forward into the unknown of the future."

Complementing Herrera's stages of mourning, Pam England describes the birth story evolution as walking through nine gates that can encompass a spectrum of narrative. Beginning with no story in the hours after birth, a mother may then start the story of relief and gratitude that her baby was born. Eventually the story shifts towards a focus on relationships during the birth: Which midwife was supportive? Which nurse was dismissive?

"Next is the medical story to rationalize why a cesarean was needed," says England. "The medical story helps prove to the mother, and anyone listening, that the cesarean was the right choice, the only way the birth could have happened." Following the medical story is the victim/judge level of birth story-telling. This is the place where most people get stuck. It's common for an HBC mother to feel like a victim from poor care management, lack of choices, and inadequate support. Victimhood is a natural place for mothers to go after a difficult or traumatic birth, and it is a striking commonality among HBC mothers.

"It's a revolving door of trauma," says England. "The victim will say 'this happened to me,' and the judge will say, 'you didn't do enough.'" In this situation, the judge can be the mother or another person. A friend might say something like, "Sometimes first-time moms have trouble relaxing enough to surrender to birth." Though malice is probably not intended, a vulnerable HBC mother can interpret this well-meaning comment as confirmation that she did something wrong. Her internal feelings of failure can trap her in a cycle of self-blame or victimhood, making it difficult to heal from her HBC.

Through time, self-work, and support from family and friends, mothers walk through the birth story gates. The final healing story according to England, "is when a mom doesn't have a need to share the details. She is a warrior, surviving her birth, and she is then able to become a teacher, a writer, a healer, and birth story listener. She has the capacity to give medicine to others."

Sharing a difficult birth story, even one that the mother has transformed into a powerful tale, may still cause her to feel uncomfortable because of the intensity of the experience. Her voice may tremble, she may feel unsafe, and the story may continue to be a trigger. If she never fully discharged the stored energy from the stress response, she will still feel anxious when she tells her story. Mothers can identify when the telling of the birth story holds power over them by tuning into subtle body changes like stomach tightness, sweating, forehead or jaw tension, or nervous energy.

I get upset and uncomfortable telling my story because I'm a doula and I wasn't meant to "fail" at my birth. Professionally, I'm supposed to be a birth leader and an example for moms.
—AMY (2002/CS, 2004/RCS, 2011/HBC; NORTHEASTERN U.S.)

As a way to cultivate a healthy birth story, midwife Ingrid Andersson asks mothers to identify what is most empowering for them when they tell their story, and what pieces they are willing to discard. Relinquishing disenfranchising moments in their births, or letting go of unenforceable rules around birth, allows a woman the space to move into a story that supports a healthy outlook on her HBC. If a mother is proud that she was able to push at the birth center before needing to transport, that can become an aspect she can highlight. If she is grateful that she tried everything she knew at the time to turn her baby from breech to head down, and from there she begins to identify more strong moments, she may be able to let go of some of the disempowering ones as well.

I've always been able to find pride in trusting my instinct to transport when I felt something was wrong. I'm proud I carried both babies to term and went into labor on my own. I wear a badge of honor after laboring over 24 hours both times to give my children the legend of a mother who fights to the end to give them her best.
—SARA (2011/HBC, 2013/CS; NORTHEASTERN U.S.)

The internal story

What is true for many mothers is that the story they tell others and the version they tell themselves are often different. It could be that a mother's internal story is one of failure, blame, self-loathing, and victimhood, while her external story is full of medical details, contraction lengths, and kindness from others. Over time, and after mothers begin personal healing through therapy, acupuncture, energy work, or other alternative modalities, their internal and external stories will begin to align. When the internal and external birth stories match, a mother is more at peace with her birth, and the story becomes a tale of motherhood and strength, where many of the details that were vital in the early months are no longer mentioned.

I told myself I failed. Most of my friends couldn't handle my grief, so the only story I told people was that I was sad. My story slowly, so slowly, shifted. I stayed in my grief until I found people who could handle it. They were people in almost the same grief as my own, other HBC women. Once I found community, my story shifted from failure, to struggle, to not-quite triumph but strength. Ultimately, I'm still a bit sad but grateful for this opportunity to find more compassion, spirit, and wisdom.
—SUE (2010/HBC, WESTERN U.S.)

My internal story involved me being a profound and terrifying failure. It was one of regret and validation that I was never going to be a good enough mother. The external story I told was that I was okay with the birth. I needed to emphasize how long I was in labor because it made me seem heroic and deflected questions about whether I'd done enough or been duped into a c-section.

I said that he needed us to go in and get him, like a child at a slumber party who calls late at night and wants to come home. People liked that analogy and I kind of did too. But it wasn't something I believed in as much as I said I did.

Now, I'm much more honest, and it's easier because I've done a lot of healing. My story still brings me pain, but it brings me joy too. It's a real story filled with everything a woman goes through as a mother, all in a very small timeframe—love, fear, expectation, survival. I'm prouder now about my birth story. It has made me who I am and it gave me a crash course in self-compassion.
—ANN (2011/HBC, MIDWESTERN U.S.)

Psychotherapist Karen Jackson Forbes says, "Healing from trauma is coming to a place where you can say, 'it's not what I wanted, but we are okay, and I forgive myself and everyone else for what happened.'" But when a mother is unable to reconcile her opposing stories because of unclear medical details, broken relationships with the birth team, or other personal reasons, self-forgiveness and absolution are tall orders.

Sometimes a woman is not ever able to accept the outcome of her birth. When this occurs, it may be helpful for her to identify her unenforceable rules around out-of-hospital birth, such as "homebirth is the safest way to birth" or "cesarean causes lifelong problems," and consider how these rules define her as a woman, mother, friend, and partner. For some women, this could be a step needed to begin challenging their pre-cesarean ideals about what successful birth means. Once their unenforceable rules around out-of-hospital birth are examined, women can begin to tease apart the story they constructed about why they should have had a home or birth center birth.

> Acknowledging what happened does not make it right. It makes it real, and dealing with those feelings and emotions are important to healing. Forgiveness is the best gift I can give myself. If I can forgive myself and the hospital staff for what happened, then I can heal.
> —Amy (2002/CS, 2004/RCS, 2011/HBC; Northeastern U.S.)

An HBC woman's healing is her next journey into discovering herself as a mother. With the support of others, she is the only one who can midwife herself into the richness of her experience, and it is her right to define the timeline she needs to do so. By being gentle with her emotional pain, she does the hard work to find peace. Women's health physical therapist Tami Lynn Kent says, "Women heal when they are ready. It's important for women to recognize that even though the homebirth cesarean happened, her healing is her responsibility, her opportunity to empower her mothering experience. Every woman will have difficult points along her mothering path, yet when she brings healing to these painful places she makes medicine for herself and her child for this life journey."

The cesarean anniversary

Though a mother may do intensive healing around her difficult birth, the cesarean anniversary can make her feel like she is losing ground in her emotional wellbeing. While some mothers have fleeting thoughts about their HBC anniversary, most describe their child's early birthdays as both a celebration and a day of secretive deep sadness.

Birth trauma peer counselor Heather Barson advises mothers to acknowledge their full range of emotions—from guilt to fear to pain—on the HBC anniversary. "It's okay to be madly in love with your children and hate the day they were born. When you're celebrating their birthday, give yourself permission to cry."

The first few birthdays after my cesarean were challenging. Not only had my plans for a homebirth been ruined and a wrench thrown into my family size planning, but I experienced a medication reaction that was extremely traumatic. It was the anniversary of meeting my baby but also the anniversary of the single most horrific event I'd ever experienced. It was hard to reconcile that and find a way to celebrate my baby without feeling re-victimized.

I felt like a traitor to my heart if I met that day with complete celebration and a traitor to my son if I allowed my own grief to creep into my reflections on his life. It took me a while to separate his birthday from my trauma, but eventually it happened. The biggest factors were time and setting the intention to help me understand them as two separate aspects of an event.

—CHRISTY (1996, 2000/HOSPITAL BIRTH, 2001/HBC, 2007/HBAC; SOUTHERN U.S.)

I take a moment throughout those three days I was in labor to pause and think about where I was, and hopefully marvel at my own strength.

—BETH (2009/HBC, WESTERN U.S.)

Crying is easy for me and I gave into it as much as I could while being strong for everyone else. I was aware that I had major healing work to do and wondered how many other mothers relive their traumatic births through gritted teeth as children toddle off with first birthday cake smeared on their cheeks.

At two, I walked through those four days of the labor anniversary laughing about how long it was. Could I really have been in labor that whole time?

Between two and three, the story of my daughter's birth began to lose its control over me and to blend into the landscape, rich in stories of motherhood. I slowly felt triumphant and brave for having worked so hard and surviving surgery with some resilience.

But three hit hard. I planned on patiently, and without judgment, seeing what came up for me. I just wept most of the days. After her birthday, I felt much better and have been able to do a lot of writing about the birth. My healing continues.

—SUE (2010/HBC, WESTERN U.S.)

The only way the anniversary is noted each year is with celebration. This day belongs to my son and we celebrate his arrival into the world and into our lives. I don't feel differently on his birthday than I do on the birthdays of his siblings (twins in 1982).

—PIPER (1982/HB, 1987/HBC; MEXICO)

HBC mother Ann posted this request to the online HBC community:

During my labor I felt so alone. It seems that many of us find our way here asking for solidarity and extra hugs on our birth anniversaries. So I want to offer and ask for something, maybe even start an informal tradition. Would anyone in this group want to be my birth anniversary partner? If so, you light a candle for me today and extinguish it the morning I gave birth. Send me a photo of the candle with a note of encouragement. On your birth anniversary, I'll do the same for you.

Women from around the world lit candles, took photos, and shared them online for Ann. Other HBC mothers checked on Ann throughout the three-day anniversary of her labor and offered support. By reaching out, Ann felt the love and connection of other women and moved through her second cesarean anniversary with community and understanding.

The gifts of the homebirth cesarean

The crossing of the HBC threshold represents the death of an innocent woman and the birth of a wise mother. With this metamorphosis, the lessons are plenty. Pam England suggests that the death of the homebirth dream eventually makes way for something new: "That doesn't come right away. It can happen months or years later, and there has to be a space made for it." Some women may gain a broader perspective about what successful birth means, compassionate understanding about other women's choices in childbirth, or personal life skills that could never have been learned without walking through the fire of an HBC.

There is real power in finding your way out of the treacherous depths of soul-sucking pain. I was able to question my core beliefs about who I am and what defines me as a woman and mama. I learned to let go of many preconceived notions of how things should be and to accept and love my attempts, knowing the path is more important than its end.

My partner also provided a gift in the way she was truly open to whatever might happen with her own homebirth, years after my HBC. Instead of letting my experience scare her, she turned it into a story of triumph. In that way, she supported me by simply taking care of herself and being such a fine example of grace and gentleness during her own pregnancy and birth.

—WENDY (2009/HBC, 2013/BORN TO PARTNER/TRANSPORT; WESTERN U.S.)

This birth made me better. I am now who I was always supposed to be.
—BETH (2009/HBC, WESTERN U.S.)

The compassion I now have for other people and the birth outreach I'm involved in almost makes my HBC experience worth it.
—ALEXIS (2011/HBC, MIDWESTERN U.S.)

I know in my heart that interventions like cesarean exist for situations like mine. In the end, the biggest gift my HBC gave me was life—mine and my son's. And for that I have huge amounts of gratitude.
—MARIZA (2011/HBC, MIDWESTERN U.S.)

Allowing the gifts from the homebirth cesarean experience to enter into daily life requires a woman shifting out of a victimhood mindset into one of compassion and openness. Maya abdominal therapist Corrine Porterfield says that "when a mother is eventually able to walk away from her birth seeing the abundance and lessons learned, she can take those treasures forward in her life. For healing to occur, it's vital she doesn't get stuck in the story and the disappointment of the birth. In the end, it's everyone finding themselves."

Relationship with the natural birth community
As women discover their personal gifts from their HBC, they are also learning how to harmonize with their natural birth communities. From nearly every woman interviewed, we heard how they felt like they no longer belonged to the homebirth and natural birthing communities, that by moving to the hospital, they lost the possibility of joining the homebirth "club." This feeling of exclusion may be caused by mothers holding shame about their births or projecting their own self-doubt as judgment from others. They may also feel scared to take the risk of speaking about their homebirth cesareans, only to be met with silence if another HBC mother is not in the room. If homebirth cesareans are rarely talked about or celebrated in the natural birth community, HBC mothers may feel no one can relate to them or that people don't want to hear their experiences.

HBC mothers are often left with a general sense of distrust and tentativeness that can be a result of not just the cesarean birth but also the stew of grief, loss, and other postpartum challenges. Everything an HBC mother has to contend with—the loss of her homebirth dream, the way she was treated by her birth team or hospital staff, her incision, her physical and mental health—compounds her fears, isolation, and sadness. This can result in her viewing the homebirth community as an insurmountable obstacle, a point of view she would not have if she were otherwise feeling emotionally healthy.

Erin Erdman runs a homebirth group and reports that when HBC mothers do return to the community they often ask permission to still participate. "These moms feel they aren't allowed to be included in the homebirth community," says Erdman. "In the group, we don't hear about the HBC experience because the moms who were part of the community when they were pregnant rarely come back after their births. They just disappear off the radar and there isn't any support for them." Erdman speculates that some women are unsure how to approach HBC mothers, especially if they had a homebirth themselves. Perhaps mothers who did give birth out-of-hospital may worry they might offend or say the wrong thing to the grieving mother, and they refrain from approaching and connecting with her.

If an HBC mother chooses not to participate with her in-person or online birth communities, it could be that she feels abandoned by the homebirth ideology in general—maybe she feels she chose an out-of-hospital birth as a safeguard against cesarean or believed that avoiding doctors would protect her from surgical birth. Some mothers may also have a sense that their natural birth community will judge them for their homebirth cesarean experience.

> *I felt less than human when talking to people from the homebirth community. They looked at my birth like a puzzle to be solved. They asked questions and dissected my experience trying to figure out what I'd done wrong, what I could have done differently. That judgment, along with my own pain, meant I cut off my local connections to that community because I was too fragile to deal with the questioning.*
> —LEAH (2012/HBC, WESTERN U.S.)

> *I felt like my birth was so off the radar of what anyone could relate to, I couldn't bring myself to attend the local new mom's group.*
> —BRANDY (2011/HBC, MIDWESTERN U.S.)

I felt like I had to constantly tell every birth detail to my homebirth friends so they would know that I did relax, that I did focus, and I tried acupuncture, and I surrendered, and I believed in my body. But I still ended up with an HBC.
—BECKY (2009, 2012/HBC; NORTHEASTERN U.S.)

No one wants to talk about homebirths that don't end at home. And no one wants to talk about midwives who don't take emotional care of their HBC clients. My midwife did what she needed to do in terms of clinical and transfer protocols, but I needed more emotional support from her. She really did abandon me emotionally, and no one in the natural birth world wants to hear about that. Homebirth is under attack and people feel that any outcome that doesn't result in a rainbow and unicorn homebirth is bad politically for midwives. But what about improving homebirth for moms who end up with cesareans? Where does that fit in?
—CARA (2005, 2007/HB, 2008/HBC; WESTERN U.S.)

Changing the conversation

It is a delicate balance for mothers and childbirth professionals to champion out-of-hospital birth and still celebrate homebirth cesareans. Welcoming HBC mothers back into the homebirth club involves open conversation about homebirths that end in cesarean. Bethany, an HBC mother, believes that by speaking up and becoming part of the narrative, HBC mothers can change the way the natural childbirth community views homebirth cesareans. But this level of comfort around HBC requires midwives, doulas, and childbirth educators to openly share HBC journeys, posting them on their websites, and inviting HBC mothers to speak at their functions. Birth expert Sarah Buckley, MD, says, "It's really important that HBC mothers come back to the natural birth community and share their stories. We must find the space to have an open dialogue so we can hear everyone's experience."

I will never be invited back to share my experience in the childbirth class I took because they don't want pregnant women to hear my kind of birth story. My story isn't posted on my midwives' website even though I could write a version they could be proud of. It would show that cesarean does happen and that it is valid. Moms could read it and critically think about that possibility. If moms never hear about HBC from their midwife, they may never think about it happening to them.
—ALEXIS (2011/HBC, MIDWESTERN U.S.)

It sucks that there are people in the natural birthing community who aren't challenged on their thinking when they reject HBC mothers as being unworthy, simply for having birth complications that excluded us from completing birth at home. We need to keep asserting our place at the homebirth table and not allow people to characterize us negatively just because they were lucky to birth at home.

—BETH (2009/HBC, WESTERN U.S.)

While the Internet is a common place to begin sharing HBC stories, posting identifying birth announcements over social media outlets such as Facebook is a gray area for birth professionals when it comes to client confidentiality. If midwives and doulas decide to publicly share information after a birth, they must be inclusive and post a range of experiences, not just "successful" homebirth stories. Birth professionals can prenatally check with clients about their comfort level in having public announcements made after their birth and explain how they handle such posts. When this is discussed prenatally, an HBC mother is less likely to assume her midwife or doula is withholding her story as a way to shame or omit the HBC experience, when in reality the birth team may just want to protect her privacy.

When the natural birth community predominately shares the "ideal" home-birth story, one where a baby is gently birthed at home, that story becomes the fact of homebirth. If that is the only way we talk about out-of-hospital births, and the only type of homebirth story we honor enough to curate in our social media feeds, blogs, and books, the shame around homebirth cesarean will continue to grow. If midwives and doulas begin posting HBC stories on their websites, childbirth educators start teaching about home-birth cesarean, and HBC mothers are invited to share their stories at home-birth socials, the darkness around HBC will dissipate.

Stories matter because stories are the facts of people's lives.

—SISTER MORNINGSTAR, CPM, MIDWESTERN U.S.

I didn't have the kind of story my midwife would ever put on her website. I didn't share my experience on my homebirth email group because it didn't fit their narrative. It was outside the bounds of a happy, empowering homebirth. My story was silent inside me, festering and bound by shame.

—ANN (2011/HBC, MIDWESTERN U.S.)

I have such a strong desire for our experiences to be included in the birth community as empowering. I feel like the movement against the medicalization of birth has gone too far the other way by labeling successful birth as a pure bliss moment, leaving no room for the pain and hardships that can, and often do, accompany birth. Maybe somewhere in the middle between this notion of a candlelit, orgasmic birth, and the planned c-section with a tummy tuck, homebirth cesarean can be included.

—JESSICA (2010/CS, 2012/HBC; SOUTHERN U.S.)

It's essential to appreciate that we are in a class different from other homebirthers. We're the ones who heard the comments about homebirth being a bad idea to begin with, then we have to defend it even though it didn't actually work for us. Most people don't understand that this type of birth shakes your faith in yourself. I don't belong to the homebirth community and am forever excluded from the homebirth club. Now when I hear the natural birth people talk about homebirth, it feels naïve. It's good to be pro-homebirth, but it needs to be tempered with pro-birth and mother supported.

—CARRIE (2011/HBC, WESTERN U.S.)

Paying close attention to how we describe out-of-hospital and cesarean births helps change the dialogue around empowered birth. HBC mother Sue once attended a talk on homebirth given by the founder of an accredited midwifery school. During the presentation, the founder shared a quote from a midwife: "If you can poop, you can birth a baby at home."

"Well, I shit every day," says Sue. "And I labored for three days trying to birth my baby at home and I couldn't do it. Even if she'd used the words *most* or *always,* it would have softened the blow." There are no guarantees in birth, and while most low-risk mothers will give birth out-of-hospital, not all will. Welcoming the full array of homebirth experiences into the natural birth conversation will usher out shame and judgment and lead to emotionally and mentally healthier mothers.

I refer to my HBC as a successful homebirth. We were at home making beautiful memories and enduring transformative pain and hardship for thirty hours. Then we went to the hospital and for twenty more hours, I succeeded in hospital birth. We tried all that we could, I pushed and pushed, and that experience brought us all closer together. Then for our last two hours, we had a successful cesarean. My baby came out safely, I endured what I never thought I could, and my husband was born into a father and partner in a way he never dreamed of.

—LEAH (2012/HBC, WESTERN U.S.)

Mothers, birth professionals, and the natural birth community have the power to change the conversation about homebirth cesareans so our daughters will see a stronger, more robust picture of empowered birth. This change begins in our hearts and scars, and spreads to our news feeds, websites, and our conversations.

Birth Professionals' Quick Guide to Changing the Conversation

- With client approval, publicly share all types of birth announcements, including homebirth cesareans.

- Welcome HBC mothers into the natural birth community.

- Create an open dialog about birth that includes homebirth cesareans.

- Be aware of language around homebirth and catchy slogans about childbirth.

- Post HBC birth stories on your websites and blogs. Share the HBC experience in your childbirth classes and at appointments.

Birth Story: Birthing a Warrior

WRITTEN BY: SARA MELONE

I never wanted a hospital birth. The hospital is where I had my tonsils removed, where my broken leg was set, where my father died. Birth didn't fit there. We would forgo the sterility of a hospital in favor of a gentle transition from peaceful womb to peaceful home.

During our first midwife visit, I relished seeing my baby's gestational sac, the tiny flicker of a heartbeat, and the light in my husband's eyes as he caught his first glimpse of our unborn child. Apart from the joy of seeing our baby, we left feeling disillusioned. Staff members were inattentive and disorganized. We were uninsured, and the fees eclipsed our mortgage. On top of that, it felt invasive discussing weight, sexual history, and pap smears with strangers. It seemed wrong inviting others into such an intimate moment. It seemed like we should birth our baby at home, alone.

So for nine months I monitored my blood pressure, measured my fundal height, and tracked my weight. I took vitamins, continued jogging, ate healthy, and tested my urine for protein. I conferred with midwife acquaintances. Two more ultrasounds revealed a lovely boy with a perfect heartbeat and no anomalies.

Knowing the rate of demise for post-date babies, I was relieved to start labor at 42 weeks. My husband timed contractions while I monitored the baby. I breathed. I visualized. I swayed. I floated in warm water. I squatted. I vocalized. I pushed. I prayed. I begged.

After four days, exhaustion swallowed me whole. Closing my eyes for a second, I'd dream a lifetime. I wanted to run away, hide in the woods, but leaving my tub of warm water meant incomprehensible pain. Each contraction hurled my body from within like a buoy bobbing at sea in gale force winds. He was mal-positioned. I had to do the thing I wanted most to avoid.

I never packed a hospital bag and left the house with only a blanket around my shoulders. I forgot my records, and the hospital stamped my chart with "no prenatal care." As they lectured me on homebirth dangers, I wanted to scream but couldn't. Following a hopeful 12-hour vigil on pitocin, I remained silent when they said "still 5" and "c-section," quietly mourning the loss of our independent birth and lamenting that the irrevocable damage of cesarean would compromise my womb forever.

We took a moment, just us two for the last time, before surrender. I cried the second he emerged, felt my heart lurch when I heard his voice, but could only lie inert while he cried in a stranger's hands. Too weak to protest his swift removal to the nursery, his indignant face appeared over the curtain only a moment before I was alone, sinking under the weight of anesthesia while the surgeons struggled to stop my bleeding. Fighting the urge to drift away, holding on for him, my body shook violently for an hour until he finally came to my arms and gazed knowingly into my eyes. We lived blissfully wrapped up in each other for less than 48 hours. Then the baby I'd planned never to be away from was taken from my arms and driven to a hospital 55 miles away for heart surgery. With no time to mourn the loss of my dream birth, I hauled my broken body up, drove through rush-hour traffic into the city, and hobbled to his bedside.

My IV had blown out three veins. I had magnesium, a blood transfusion, and a horrible incision. Arriving at his bedside, I was dismayed to see my formerly unscathed newborn on an IV. After surgery he had magnesium, a blood transfusion, and a fresh incision on his perfect little body. I was devastated, but infinitely proud of my little warrior. We fought through the same war and came out with matching battle scars.

Back home, I was unsure how I could ever birth again, but trusted I would feel different in a few years. Conceiving 6 ½ months later was surreal. When an ultrasound foretold another boy, I broke down, fearing the same events would unfold. I'd done everything to secure a healthy natural birth the first time and still wound up in the OR. I felt powerless.

Then somewhere in the panic, I remembered a precious new life that required celebration. Another ultrasound confirmed what we inexplicably knew in our hearts—we were actually having a girl. In that moment, I experienced an awakening. It was a different baby, a different pregnancy. History need not repeat. I am strong, never powerless.

I started chiropractic and belly binding to tuck her into my pelvis. I drank red raspberry leaf tea, took pulsatilla and evening primrose oil. I bounced on a yoga ball and processed lingering doubts within the supportive environment of the online HBC group. I met with both an OB and a midwife in an attempt to marry my holistic homebirthing heart with my high-risk hospital birth reality. And I wrote a birth plan for hospital staff with two sections: one for VBAC, and one for cesarean.

When her February 12th due date came and went, I knew she was waiting for Valentine's Day. I woke with contractions at 2 AM the morning of the 14th and spent the day in a labor of love before heading to the hospital.

As Valentine's Day came to a close, everything came to a head. At eight centimeters, her heart rate was questionable. My attending doctor vanished to perform another patient's cesarean on the heels of prepping me to "get ready" to submit to cesarean. I asked to change my position to help her descend, I asked for an explanation of their concern, and I asked for more time. When the on-call doctor scoffed at my suggestions, accused me of illogical thinking, and declared I wanted to be "in control"—with the implication that participating in my own medical care was somehow wrong—I asked her to stop. I asked her to remember that her patient was a woman and a mother with real emotions, trying to make the healthiest decisions for her children.

Because I chose a hospital supportive of skin-to-skin in the OR, I was horrified to be told my baby would be taken for evaluation. I shook my head, speechless. The surgeon assured me it would only be a few minutes. I refused. I told her they could evaluate the baby while she was on my chest, that I was separated from my son at birth, and they wouldn't take another baby from me.

Signing surgical consent forms was like signing my own death warrant. Feeling stripped of humanity, I said nothing as hands shuttled my body through the surgical assembly line like a carcass. I thought of my son sleeping down the hall, praying he wouldn't awaken and cry for me while I was immobilized. My husband's fingertips on my head felt comforting, but I couldn't even look at him. Staring at the ceiling in mute despair, I wondered how I could do this again, but knew I somehow would. After everything I suffered the first time—the death of a dream, my surgery, his surgery, our awful separation and broken hearts—I already knew there is nothing I won't do for the beautiful babies who chose me to be their mother. I'd walk through fire for them. These births were my fire. I'd gone in a scared pregnant woman, but a fierce mother had been cast out of the molten steel born inside those flames.

Momentary disgust and disbelief washed over me as the doctor opened me, declared my uterine scar was separating, and told me I'd made a "good choice." I shut everything out until my daughter's furious cry broke the quiet and brought me to tears. I called out for her, snatched her from their hands, and held her tight. She was pink and smelled of sweet vernix. She peed all over my neck, and I was never so happy.

It's not easy being a cesarean mama, but I realize now there's no right or wrong way to birth, only different ways. Like life, birth is imperfect, wild, and unpredictable. I don't expect life to be perfect, but I somehow thought birth should be. I'd pursued a kind of fairytale that isn't always attainable. In some ways it seems fitting. Creating life is so substantial, we shouldn't be allowed passage through this sacred rite without giving from some place. For me, it was humble surrender of the ideal birth I required and lying down to birth in the way that was required of me.

I'm not lucky in birth. I'm blessed in other ways. I conceived two healthy pregnancies without morning sickness or complication. Two years later, my milk nourishes two children who are exactly as I envisioned, the loveliest parts of their parents. They adore each other, make me laugh, and challenge me to be my best. I'll always be disappointed I can't birth how I want, but I choose to focus on the blessings I do have. The moment of birth is one out of millions—a moment no more definitive than the thousands before or after. My children are not ruined for their birth, so I cannot be either.

Chapter 12

Slaying the dragon

After nearly five days of labor, the doctor told me it was time to call a c-section. While everyone was thinking of the baby in my womb, I was the only one also thinking of babies still to come. Every future child would be affected by this cesarean, and our family size might be dictated by surgical birth risks. The cesarean was already taking away my freedom of choice before we'd even gotten to the operating table.

Birthing a second time seemed unfathomable, but six months after my HBC, a faint pink line appeared on a pregnancy test. "Oh shit. Dear God, I'm not ready for birth again." Then a calm came over me. Maybe this is my chance to have a different birth, to regain the faith I'd lost. But what will that mean? Will I love this baby more if the birth goes "right"? What if it's another cesarean? Will I be angry and wonder why that would happen to me?
—SARA (2011/HBC, 2013/CS; NORTHEASTERN U.S.)

For HBC mothers, the ripple effect on future childbearing is tremendous. Some women choose not to have more children because the pain caused by their first homebirth cesarean was unbearable, and the idea of repeating that experience is unthinkable. Others felt that their physical and mental recovery was too rough and make the decision to not have any more children, even though they were previously open to it. On the other end of the spectrum, women may welcome the opportunity to prove to themselves that they are capable of birthing a baby vaginally or hope that the next birth will bring a sense of resolution to unanswered questions. This chapter explores the personal decision-making process about family size; the doubts, fears, and choices that arise during subsequent pregnancies; and the gut-wrenching emotional evolution that takes place after another HBC.

The decision process

Women who have had HBCs usually go through a deeply personal exploration of their intentions surrounding future births. For some women, the trauma from their HBC is too deep—physically, emotionally, or both, and the possibility of birthing another child no longer exists. This is true for women who feel they cannot mentally survive another childbirth experience, and those who might have special scars that prohibit a safe pregnancy.

> *Because of my emotional difficulty around the HBC, we will never, ever have another biological child.*
> —Carol (2012/HBC, Western U.S.)

For women who know that their families are complete at one child, their grief takes on a particular quality of loss. For these women it's important that they are able to reclaim their confidence and power in ways that do not focus on achieving a future vaginal birth.

> *My midwife said I can try for a VBAC and I remember thinking this is the only child we want to have, so no, I won't get another at-bat. There is a small part of me that wants to have another shot at birth, to maybe grab the prize I didn't get the first time. But for now, another child means a do-over of birth and that's not something I'm comfortable with.*
> —Ann (2011/HBC, Midwestern U.S.)

Many HBC women question their inclination for more children as a possible hidden agenda for a "successful" birth, one where they are able to push their babies out of their vaginas. This wishful thinking can lead a woman towards trying to conceive or it can be enough to make her resist the urge to conceive again.

For families who choose to have another child, the vacillation, fears, and questions without answers are all part of the decision process. HBC parents face greater emotional, physical, and labor risk factors than before their homebirth cesareans. Logistically, mothers now have to contend with the additional risk factors that pregnancy and labor present after a surgical birth. The legal status of midwives attending a VBAC and insurance coverage for attempting a VBAC must be considered along with the grueling decision of possibly scheduling another cesarean. Emotionally, HBC mothers need to find supportive care providers; handle potential triggers during pregnancy, labor, birth, and postpartum; and deal with friends and family who may be angry or uncomfortable with their choices.

> *My state required a minimum of 18 months between births in order for a midwife to legally attend an HBAC. My children would be 15 months apart, so my choice on birth location was made for me.*
> —SARA (2011/HBC, 2013/CS; NORTHEASTERN U.S.)

Trust and relationships after an HBC

A pregnancy following a homebirth cesarean can stir powerful emotions and force women to re-examine relationships with family and friends, the natural birth community, and even their partners. For a mother whose family and friends were unsupportive after her HBC, she may be reluctant to discuss her birth choices with them. Fearing judgment, she may feel unready to answer questions about where and how she will birth the next time around.

> *I can say with confidence that out of my family, I was the most informed about childbirth, but I was treated as though I was utterly ignorant and uninformed because of my choices. Although their concern came from love, all it did was pile on so much stress that I ended up physically ill. Next time, I won't be discussing my plans with them.*
> —EMMA (2012/HBC, AUSTRALIA)

Relationships between the mother and her birth team can also be tested. The local midwifery community is usually small, making out-of-hospital care options geographically limited. A mother who had a negative experience with a midwife may have undesirable choices available when seeking care during her next pregnancy. If the mother needs to engage the hospital system again, she may awaken powerful triggers and be reluctant to even attend prenatal appointments with an OB/GYN. This could cause her to feel isolated and disconnected from her baby and her highest intention for the birth.

> *When we began thinking of a second child, I was apprehensive about trying to find a new midwife because I know that the homebirth community is tightly knit. I was also slightly nervous that our first midwife might hear of our pregnancy and try to contact me to patch things up.*
> —ALLIE (2010/HBC, 2012/HBAC; MIDWESTERN U.S.)

If a partner did not provide adequate support during the HBC or more commonly, during the postpartum time, that relationship may be strained. Ideally, HBC couples agree to face feelings of guilt, failure, and difficult negotiations with each other before they become pregnant again. If they aren't willing to engage with each other about their emotional wounds, they may be unable to find resolution before moving forward to a new birth.

> My HBC hasn't deterred me from wanting another child, but it has changed some of the details. It was very upsetting talking about future pregnancies because I felt a loss of autonomy since my husband would only agree to a repeat c-section. And it was heartbreaking to see the intense fear in his eyes when we discussed alternatives.
> —LEAH (2012/HBC, WESTERN U.S.)

A mother's trust in her partner can be challenged after her HBC, and that can significantly play into her next birth. She may worry that her partner will "give up" on her during labor or in the event of another unwanted outcome, that her partner will be unable to support her emotionally.

> My husband promised he wouldn't let them force me into any interventions, but he caved as soon as the doctor said cesarean. How can I ever trust him again?
> —RACHEL (2013/HBC, WESTERN U.S.)

The HBC experience can be scary for partners who relinquish control to the natural forces of labor and are met with a birth that falls outside of their expectations.

> With our first child, I treated pregnancy like a high school assignment: I did just enough prep to get by at the expense of accurate information. This resulted in me supporting a bad medical call just because an OB advised it. Next time, I want to educate myself rather than trusting the providers and following whatever they tell me.
> —ERIC, PARTNER OF RACHEL (2013/HBC, WESTERN U.S.)

> I don't think another birth could even be close to as bad as the first, and I'm not worried about it. The HBC changed a lot about what I know about birth, but not the way I view birth.
> —LEE, PARTNER OF LAUREN (2011/HBC, SOUTHERN U.S.)

Our HBC was stressful and traumatic for both of us, but it feels like a distant memory to me now. I know my wife has a very different perspective on that and is still haunted and traumatized by her experience. My trepidation about having another child has more to do with what comes after—feeling overwhelmed, the lack of time for myself, all the usual stresses of parenting that don't hit home until you actually experience them.
—JACKSON, PARTNER OF DAISY (2007/HBC, NORTHEASTERN U.S.)

I tend to withdraw when the topic of more kids comes up. I know Serra wants to plan a homebirth, but I'm not sure I can handle that. What if we have to transport again? How will I take care of her mental health and two children when we don't have any family in town to help us?
—KELLY, PARTNER OF SERRA (2010/HBC, WESTERN U.S.)

I wanted two kids and we talked about that before the HBC, but I knew the minute she went into surgery that she would not want another child. In that moment, I accepted it. It felt like a door slamming shut and it wasn't my place to knock on that door.
—DAVE, PARTNER OF COURTNEY (2011/HBC, WESTERN U.S.)

Similar to healing from a difficult birth, mothers and partners can work together to support and honor each other's differences with open communication and mutual respect. Listening without blame and sharing each other's birth story perspectives are ways to build communication focused on subsequent births. During this sharing, a mother may be surprised to hear that her partner thought she was strong and powerful during her HBC. Likewise a partner may learn that he was passively appreciated by the mother in the weeks following the birth. If each person can try to identify at least one moment during the HBC that was positive, an occasion where they admired their partner or a time where they recall both being intimately connected with each other, it could go a long way towards healing.

Intimacy and sex after an HBC
There is a mainstream myth that a surgical birth "saves" vaginas and that cesarean women are lucky, sexually speaking, since their vagina didn't have to stretch to accommodate a baby. However, the weight of the uterus during pregnancy can alter vaginal shape and elasticity even before labor begins. Combine that with the fact that many HBC women pushed for hours and

moved their babies low into their vaginas only to have them pulled up and out through their abdomen, possibly causing stretching, tearing, and altered mobility patterns of the pelvic bowl.

Hesitation and fears of sexual intimacy in the time following birth are a common challenge for many postpartum couples, even those that birthed vaginally—they are tired, stressed, and most likely don't have much of a sex drive. Postpartum and lactation hormones can make sex uncomfortable, and feelings about a changed body after pregnancy can make sex a low priority or even intolerable.

What separates this issue from vaginal birthing mothers is that many HBC women connect their lack of libido, reluctance to sexually engage, or painful intercourse to their stressful or traumatic HBCs. They described feeling paralyzed with memories of the cesarean when trying to have sex, and sometimes they find that lying on their backs is difficult, since it is reminiscent of lying on the operating table and having their bodies exposed and touched. Women also reported continually thinking about their scar when intimate with their partners, and sometimes a mere graze of a partner's hand on the scar would shut down a woman's arousal. HBC-related guilt and shame impede women's sexual feelings, while adhesions and tissue congestion in the pelvic bowl caused from surgery can result in painful sex and intercourse.

> I labored throughout our apartment and every room reminded me of the ambulance transport. It wasn't until we moved to a new home that I was able to become sexually active with my partner.
> —Uma (2006/HBC, Southern U.S.)

> Fifteen months out and sex is not even on the table for us. I feel like it's never going to happen and what's worse, I don't care.
> —Ashley (2008/CS, 2011/HBC; Midwestern U.S.)

> I was sad to have a uterine scar rather than the typical perineal tenderness from a vaginal birth. Receiving and giving attention to that part of my body refreshed the sadness and memories of my birth. I felt as though my connection and trust with my uterus and vagina had been cut during the cesarean.
> —Terra (2011/HBC, Northeastern U.S.)

In the days following my HBC, I wanted to have sex as a way to affirm a deeper relationship. Quickly that feeling faded and we didn't have sex for a year. Anytime my husband would run his hand over my scar, or even my stomach, I would be reminded of my HBC. It would all come back when we were close—my failed womanhood, the memories of how my husband saw me after my HBC, how he cared for me in all of my uncleanliness and postpartum grossness. Then, there is my fear that our birth control will fail and I will become pregnant again. My mind, instead of focusing on the matter at hand, drifts towards birth, towards a victorious VBAC or another "failure." All of it comes to mind when we try to have sex. Just like my postpartum depression is inseparable from my HBC, so also is sex.

This was hard for my husband. We had a lot of conflicts, we grew apart, and our relationship was taxed. Once we made intimacy, although not intercourse, a thing that we needed to work on, our relationship improved greatly. We started hugging and laughing again together.

—KATE (2012/HBC, SOUTHERN U.S.)

Bryan Baisinger, DC, treats postpartum women who experience painful sex and intercourse. He says that women experiencing pain with sex have a unique mixture of physical and psychological factors that generate sexual-related pain. "Before healing really begins" says Baisinger, "loved ones, care providers, and affected women must trust they are in pain when they say they are, even when the cause is not understood." He goes on to say that one of the most common physical causes for painful sex after a cesarean is soft tissue alteration and myofascial trigger points around the scar line and in the pelvic bowl. He recommends self-care at home by gently massaging around the scar and rolling the skin between the fingers to help break up small adhesions. Seeking professional help from a qualified pelvic floor specialist can speed the healing process for most women. (See Appendix H, Physical Healing Modalities after an HBC.)

For a woman who experiences hesitation or painful sex and intercourse, going slow, listening to her body, and having a partner who is willing to engage in forms of intimacy that are not intercourse are important for building sex back into the relationship. Couples talk about feelings of contentment and pleasure when hugging, playing, and special time are a regular part of their daily lives.

When partners can view intimacy, not sex, as a needed first step toward healing, they can better understand that a woman's return to her body after a difficult birth can be a process of going slow and staying connected with each other.

> I understood how fragile and potentially triggering intimacy would be and I was prepared to be very slow and gentle. Having the opportunity to just touch her body again was a big deal, even if we didn't have sex. That feeling of closeness and intimacy never waned; it was a part of our ongoing healing. It wasn't about the act of sex, but the moment of intimacy.
>
> —DAVE, PARTNER OF COURTNEY (2011/HBC, WESTERN U.S.)

For mothers who are interested in moving forward as sexual beings, engaging in therapy, exercise to boost self-confidence, or physical and energetic healing modalities such as acupuncture and massage are ways to regain a sense of self and sexuality. Learning how to gratify themselves first, before having to focus on the needs of a partner, can be a low-pressure way for women to reclaim their bodies and sensuality.

Pregnant again

Planned or unplanned, facing a pregnancy after an HBC is likely to cause mixed emotions. All the lost dreams from the homebirth cesarean, along with fears, and consequences of the HBC, are dredged to the surface and highlighted.

> There is a sense of fear with this next birth. We know that having a cesarean is a very real possibility, but that shouldn't stop us from pushing forward to bring our next child into the world the way that we want.
>
> —DAVID, PARTNER OF MICHELE (2011/HBC, 7 WEEKS PREGNANT; WESTERN U.S.)

> Before trying to conceive, I had to reach the point that the desire to create and raise another life was greater than my fear of c-section and everything that comes with it. There's more horsepower behind giving this next baby a good birth, but I'm also more willing to sacrifice my educated idea of what a good birth entails.
>
> —MICHELE (2011/HBC, 7 WEEKS PREGNANT; WESTERN U.S.)

I'm having to ask questions, make decisions, and compromise in order to get my best chance at attempting a VBAC. It's all so much more difficult this time around, and it makes the pregnancy stressful and less exciting. I'm a little afraid that the more hope I have, the more disappointment I'll face. I need to make peace with a c-section, but I'm having great difficulty doing it. The clock is ticking for me to deal with these issues, but at the end of the day if I wind up with a c-section again, I will have a lot of emotional pain.
—JULIA (2011/HBC, 24 WEEKS PREGNANT; WESTERN U.S.)

My HBC took so much away from me but I will not let it take my son's sibling. To not have another kid would have been one more defeat. This next birth can be worse, and it'll still be worth it. If I have another HBC, I know I'll have better perspective this time. I know I'll be able to put aside my feelings of self-doubt and denial that I had with my first. This time around, I'm already a mom. And the mom in me knows I'll heal, emotionally and physically.
—ALEXIS (2011/HBC, 18 WEEKS PREGNANT; MIDWESTERN U.S.)

This time, I'll be birthing in a hospital. I still believe in homebirth, but it doesn't matter where I birth. I don't feel totally safe in the hospital. And I don't feel totally safe out-of-hospital either. I came to a realization that it isn't about a woman birthing "where she feels safest." It's about us knowing that although birth and life are completely unsafe, we can trust ourselves to handle what happens wherever we are. If this baby is born by cesarean, I won't be happy about it, but it won't destroy me. I don't NEED a VBAC. I want one and plan on fighting for it. But however this child comes into the world, we will be okay.
—BETH (2009/HBC, 19 WEEKS PREGNANT; WESTERN U.S.)

Choosing Vaginal Birth After Cesarean (VBAC)

When pregnant again, many HBC women want to try for a vaginal birth. However, some of these women do not have the option of pursuing a midwife-attended vaginal birth after cesarean (VBAC) outside of the hospital due to restrictions on midwives' scope of care. This leaves women the choice of an unassisted homebirth or attempting a VBAC in the hospital.

All hospitals place restrictions on women attempting a VBAC, but some are more favorable than others. Certain doctors may also refuse to attend VBACs for fear of malpractice, hospital protocol, or insurance issues. If allowing a trial of labor, hospital staff may set women up for disappointment by undermining her labor efforts. For example, a physician might initiate conversations during labor about uterine rupture in the hopes that she will choose the "safe" option and consent to another cesarean. Women hoping for a VBAC in the hospital can research which hospitals and providers are comfortable with VBACs, and ask about their successful VBAC rates.

> I was determined to try a VBAC. From my first prenatal visit, I was shocked by the assumptions of medical personnel that I would automatically schedule a cesarean and even more disheartened by their assessments that I was more prone to cesarean because of my height, body structure, BMI, and even my shoe size.
> —SARA (2011/HBC, 2013/CS; NORTHEASTERN U.S.)

In progressively minded communities where out-of-hospital is a more acceptable option, there are hospitals and care providers who are very supportive of VBACs. For an HBC woman who is fortunate to have access to this kind of care, her doctor or nurse midwife might understand her desires for her birth and be able to maintain an open level of communication as labor progresses. Some VBAC mothers we spoke with reported that the hospital staff was invested in their wants and strived to ensure that even in the face of a drastic change of plans, like another cesarean, these mothers had a say in their births.

An HBC mother who chooses to plan an out-of-hospital birth for her future children, either with midwives or unassisted, now has a greater understanding of the range of possibilities her birth may take. Women we interviewed said they were more prepared to address difficult conversations with their birth team, and they were clear on their own personal boundaries regarding the length of labor and the conditions under which they would transport to the hospital. They also reported dips and spikes in their confidence levels about the upcoming birth. Though these women have a more realistic idea of what labor and birth may look like, pregnancy still can be a triggering and an emotionally difficult time.

> I'm afraid that if I'm not able to VBAC, it will break me. I'm worried that if I am able to have a VBAC, it won't make me feel any better or it will make me feel worse. I feel like my confidence is shot. All I can imagine is a transport

and inevitable cesarean. I want to visualize a peaceful homebirth, but I did so much of that last time, it feels silly. I feel like a jaded woman thinking back to her silly schoolgirl dreams.
—LIBBY (2011/HBC, 33 WEEKS PREGNANT; MIDWESTERN U.S.)

Women certainly can feel victorious, healed, and elated once they experience the vaginal birth they so wanted. They may find relief in discovering they are capable of birthing vaginally after their previous HBC made them feel "broken" or inept. Many post-VBAC women reported a miraculous connection with their babies and deep gratification knowing they pushed their babies out of their bodies.

My HBAC was incredibly healing and worked wonders to ease the pain from my HBC. That was not an intentional part of my birth planning, though. It was an unplanned side effect. I always get nervous and sad when I hear a mother mention planning another baby to finally "get to have my natural birth experience." There are no guarantees in birth. It would have been hard enough had my second homebirth ended in cesarean without having put the added pressure on myself to meet some mystical and unrealistic standard of what is a "good" birth.
—CHRISTY (1996, 2000/HOSPITAL BIRTH, 2001/HBC, 2007/HBAC; SOUTHERN U.S.)

In the event of a vaginal birth after cesarean, the HBC mother might suffer feelings of guilt that she was able to birth one child in the way she wanted but not able to give her HBC child that same experience. She may have fears of unintentionally favoring one child or developing a closer mother-child bond as a result of a more ideal birth experience. It can also be tempting to attribute one child's less favorable personality traits to a more stressful mode of birth, and this can be internalized as maternal failure.

My HBC baby was terrified of people and new situations for a long time. I couldn't help but worry that his anxiety was a product of hospitals, nurses, and doctors. I was constantly reassuring him I would never let anyone hurt him, and no one would ever take him again. My second baby has always been more needy and high-maintenance. I wondered if it's because she bonded immediately after the cesarean—that I trained her to need me more. Two totally different children, but I still manage to find motherly guilt and "blame" even though they're both perfectly well-bonded with not a thing "wrong."

In the end, I made peace knowing that no matter how they were born, each child would have their own unique tale of birth. My only job as their

mother was to take the journey, embrace them, and discover the best parts of their stories.
—SARA (2011/HBC, 2013/CS; NORTHEASTERN U.S.)

Along with joy, a VBAC can also bring about additional feelings of regret concerning a previous HBC. If a VBAC proves there is nothing inherently flawed with the mother's ability to birth vaginally, then what went wrong during the HBC? What could she have done differently to ensure that her last baby had also been born "correctly"? A VBAC might even accentuate her original feelings of failure over her HBC and reinforce all those nagging *what ifs* running through her mind. For some women, the success of a VBAC manifests as an emotional let-down which may be difficult for her to understand since her greatest wish was for a vaginal birth. For those who subsequently give birth vaginally, attaining a VBAC may not provide a fix-all solution to healing the pain of an HBC.

My homebirth was great. I did it! But I have a lot of guilt in comparing my two births. I had a really hard time bonding with my HBC baby. With my homebirth baby, I knew she was mine as soon as I picked her up out of the water. I didn't get that with my first.
—MAUREEN (2009/HBC, 2012/HBAC; WESTERN U.S.)

Echoing Maureen's experience, Leah expresses concern about how a vaginal birth might affect her relationship with her HBC child:

Part of me worries that if I do succeed in having a VBAC with immediate and uninterrupted access to a new baby, my bond with that baby will be stronger than with my daughter and I'll feel guilty about my HBC or damage my relationship with her.
—LEAH (2012/HBC, WESTERN U.S.)

At 15 weeks pregnant, Libby is trying trying to cope with the same fears that Leah wonders about:

I'm worried that I'm going to bond with this baby more than I did with my son. What if the tenuous bond that I have with my son is broken and I love the new baby more?

After several days of labor at home, Libby transported to the hospital for a VBAC. She says:

> It's a relief to know that I could actually birth vaginally. But I feel terrible admitting that I feel bad after this vaginal birth because there is still a sense of loss that came with it, even though it was what I wanted. I have a picture of me holding my daughter right after she was born and I don't remember ever feeling so happy. You can see it on my face, pure bliss. It's the most beautiful picture I have of myself, but even with that absolute joy, I still feel loss. I thought the VBAC would fix me from feeling broken. It didn't. VBAC wasn't the answer.
>
> —Libby (2011/HBC, 2013/VBAC transport; Midwestern U.S.)

The message that we heard repeatedly from mothers who went on to have a vaginal birth is that healing happens between births, not because of a specific birth outcome.

Facing the HBC dragon

Experiencing another HBC may allow a woman to rediscover her inner strength by taking control of her birth the next time around. Even though she ends up in surgery, she is more prepared, not as blindsided, and usually better able to adapt to less than ideal circumstances. Often it takes the extreme powerlessness of an unexpected HBC to strengthen a mother's resolve so that she can take back her power during another surgical birth. Many women go into subsequent surgical births armed with the knowledge of cesarean practices that respect the mother's wishes.

> I felt ready for a homebirth or a cesarean. I went into my second birth with the desire to slay the dragon. I ended up not with the birth that was in my head, but one that I was more connected to. It was an amazing experience to walk away from a second HBC and feel powerful and strong. This time, feeling so differently, I know my body did a good job.
>
> Having a homebirth was never going to be the answer for me. Once I embraced that, it became a source of pride. Maybe I didn't do it your way, but you sure as hell didn't do it my way. After my births, I feel like I deserve a superhero cape.
>
> —Korin (2006, 2012/HBC; Western U.S.)

My second HBC was dramatically different from my first. When I transferred the second time, I knew what to expect, our midwife had a good relationship with the hospital, and she helped keep my mind open to all outcomes. I didn't have a huge hurdle of emotional recovery because the process didn't devastate me the way it did the first time. My second HBC still brought up self-doubt, but I was able to move myself through it more easily knowing that how my baby came into the world is not a reflection of my strength, womanhood, or ability to be a wonderful mother.
—JENNIFER (2007, 2010/HBC; WESTERN U.S.)

On the other end of the multiple-HBC spectrum are women who felt they chose a strong birth team, prepared themselves for the possibility of another HBC, tried to assert themselves in the hospital, but because of unsupportive hospital staff or circumstances that worked against them, they did not have an empowering experience.

Feeling like I knew what to expect only meant that the trauma was even more of a shock. I thought there was no way I could have two homebirth cesareans. It just didn't seem likely because I planned my birth so differently the second time.
—TOREY (2005, 2009/HBC; SOUTHERN U.S.)

Scheduling another cesarean

Another possible outcome after an HBC is that the mother could suffer a relapse of the same painful emotions she experienced with her previous HBC(s). For a woman who had multiple HBCs, she may feel more betrayed and disappointed in her body after each cesarean. It is the knowledge of this possible emotional relapse, a medical condition like placenta previa, or an acceptance that she may not have a vaginal birth that guides some women to choose a repeat cesarean (RCS).

My husband believes I don't need surgery and I can birth vaginally, but he's terribly worried that if we attempt an HBAC and end up with a c-section, it will be as devastating to me or worse than the first. He wants me to have an emotionally healthier postpartum this time around.

I'm afraid to find out I'm truly as broken as my HBC made me feel. I'm afraid to confirm that I cannot do what the female body is supposed to. I'm afraid another HBC will break my spirit—and if it does, I don't know how

to care for not one but two children. So our decision is to schedule a repeat cesarean. The idea of going into labor and failing is too much.
—HEATHER (2009/HBC, 33 WEEKS PREGNANT; MIDWESTERN U.S.)

I chose to schedule a cesarean because I tried my hardest two times to have a homebirth. The pain was excruciating both times, with both ending in cesarean. I decided that I could let myself off the hook for having to go through that pain again. I had to do a lot of healing to surrender to that decision. But by scheduling a cesarean, I could relax more about my birth the third time.
—ERIN (2007, 2009/HBC, 2011/RCS; WESTERN U.S.)

Some women may never discover if they can push a baby out of their bodies. Even if they schedule a repeat cesarean, these women may forever be haunted by the *what ifs* of labor and birth. When this is the case, women we interviewed reported that just like the healing process from their HBC, they sought professional help from therapists, acupuncturists, and other alternative body healers.

If HBC experiences have taught us anything, it is that women need to feel supported and heard, regardless of where or how they decide to birth. Along with welcoming homebirth cesareans into the natural birth community, we must support women in all their birth choices.

If I ever come to a place where I'm pregnant again and wanting another child, not just another birth, I envision scheduling a repeat cesarean. If I decide I'd like to go through birth again, I deserve what all women do, which is to make my own decisions without judgment from others. Whatever my choice, I believe it should be honored, respected, and supported by not only compassionate care providers, but by the other mothers in my life. We can never know what it's like to walk in another woman's shoes, to live with the wisdom she carries in her bones, born of her unique life experiences. Judging another woman's choices in birth is ignorant and cruel. Birth is hard enough without someone else pressing their views on us. That was true when I was criticized for planning a homebirth. It will be true if I decide never to have another child. And it will be true if I decide to schedule a repeat cesarean. What is at stake is women's right to determine how it is best for them to birth, whether it's at home, in a tub, or on an operating table.
—ANN (2011/HBC, MIDWESTERN U.S.)

It does get better:
an afterword of voices

Here we offer insight from HBC mothers, partners, and birth professionals in their own words, without narrative. Our hope is that readers will take these experiences, and the stories throughout this book, and move forward personally and professionally with greater compassion and appreciation of the homebirth cesarean experience.

To HBC mothers

There are positive lessons to be learned from an HBC. It's hard to see them initially, when you're blinded by grief, rage, and the morass of emotions, but as your healing unfolds, you can find wisdom in your experience.
—STEPHANIE (2008, 2012/HBC; NORTHEASTERN U.S.)

Find someone you can vent to, someone who doesn't mind the tears, the questions, the anger re-hashed even years later.
—LAURA (2003, 2008, 2011/HBC; MIDWESTERN U.S.)

It does get better.
—NICOLE (2011/HBC, MIDWESTERN U.S.)

You will heal, and you will forgive yourself for feeling that you failed. You will never forget, because this kind of mark runs deeper even as the scar begins to fade. In time you will realize that no matter the choices you made, you did the best you could. And in the end, you gave your child the best birth that the moment could offer—even if it wasn't the one you wished for.
—HEATHER (2009/HBC, MIDWESTERN U.S.)

It's so important to break free of the victim role and emerge into a place of empowerment. It's not healthy to hold onto anger or hatred. It's also important that we not feel ashamed or allow others to degrade our experiences.
—CHRISTINE (2009, 2012/HBC; NORTHEASTERN U.S.)

Your HBC is just one part of you. It does not have to be the only thing that defines you, although it may contribute significantly to who you are.
—PIPER   (1982/HB, 1987/HBC; MEXICO)

Maybe your baby had an awesome birth experience, even if yours was difficult. Both of those things can be true at the same time.
—ANN (2011/HBC, MIDWESTERN U.S.)

If the help you're getting isn't what you need, don't be afraid to say no to it and keep asking until you find what is helpful. Take it on as a mission to prove that you are not alone, because you can feel so isolated after an HBC. Find the people who are going to tell you that you did a good job.
—RACHEL (2009/HBC, WESTERN U.S.)

You'll find yourself progressing through stages of healing. In the beginning, that process might be dominated by numbness and grief. You'll also go through a period of anger and bitterness. Eventually, you'll work your way to acceptance, in which your HBC no longer determines how you define yourself. You'll be triggered less often and have unexpected chances to make peace with your cesarean.
—CHRISTY, (1996,2000/HOSPITAL,2001/HBC, 2007/HBAC; SOUTHERN U.S.)

To birth professionals

Choose your words carefully around cesarean. You don't know how a mom might hear them.
—LENNON CLARK, CPM, WESTERN U.S.

Educate mothers about the term HBC. Naming the birth experience is healing.
—CYNTHIA, (2012/HBC, SOUTHERN U.S.)

Birth workers must stop treating c-section like the illegitimate birth no one wants to talk about. Cesarean can be beautiful when you're prepared for it. Prepare us. And prepare yourselves to care for us afterward.
—SARA (2011/HBC, 2013/CS; NORTHEASTERN U.S.)

Support of the client shouldn't end with a transfer of care. This is when the woman needs you most, not when you walk away.
—MISTY (2008/HBC, 2011/HBAC; WESTERN U.S.)

Ask the partners what it was like for them. Remind the partner that mom will always have had that cesarean. Cesarean is not something that only lives in the past tense.
—DAVE, PARTNER OF COURTNEY (2011/HBC, WESTERN U.S.)

Midwifery is a very emotionally enriching and bonding experience with a family, and there needs to be sound judgment free of a midwife's own emotions and birth expectations. One of the midwife's jobs is to be aware of her own feelings and how they affect the relationship with the birthing family.
—JUSTIN, PARTNER OF TERRA (2011/HBC, NORTHEASTERN U.S.)

Call for backup from a fresh and rested midwife who might have new ideas when you've exhausted your tools.
—HEATHER, (1995/TRANSPORT, 2008, 2011/HBC, CPM; WESTERN U.S.)

As an HBC supporter, be calm, listen, and make space for processing like you would for a vaginal birth.
—SCARLETT LYNSKY, CHILDBIRTH EDUCATOR, WESTERN U.S.

To partners

Take care of yourself. The first month is critical to make sure you're maintaining your own sanity in a healthy way, in whatever form that takes—writing, exercising, connecting with friends.
—DAVE, PARTNER OF COURTNEY (2011/HBC, WESTERN U.S.)

You need to have as much support as possible. You and the mother both need that.
—JIM, PARTNER OF REBECCA (2012/HBC, SOUTHERN U.S.)

The mother may grieve for a very long time after the birth. Instead of trying to "make it better," practice listening—hold the space for her to express her feelings, even if it makes you uncomfortable. Understand that you may be hearing the same story repeatedly as she processes it, and be okay with that. Trying to help too actively may inadvertently cause her to feel like you don't want to hear her anymore.
—STEPHANIE (2008, 2012/HBC; NORTHEASTERN U.S.)

Hire a postpartum doula who can absorb some of the experiencing you may be feeling. This relieves the mother from feeling like she needs to shoulder your pain as well as her own and possibly the baby's. The emotional support of an experienced doula is hard to beat.
—CARISSA (2012/HBC, MIDWESTERN U.S.)

HBC mothers, you have the capacity to bring healing to women, families, and the natural birth community. In your wombs and hearts, you carry new understanding about what it means to give birth in the operating room. Trust your path. Gather around the fire, share your journey, touch your wounds. Find the strong story of your birth. What feels like the unknown, what feels scary and dark, is actually your own power, the power created from your homebirth cesarean.

APPENDIX A:

PLAN C

Plan A is a homebirth. Plan B is a vaginal birth at the hospital. Plan C is a homebirth cesarean.

—AMANDA ROE, NATUROPATHIC MIDWIFE, WESTERN U.S.

Plan C is a conversation starter and postpartum planning guide for birth professionals and expectant families. It is a tool to help prenatally introduce the possibility of a homebirth cesarean (HBC) and to expand the knowledge around what choices might be available in the event of a non-emergent surgical birth. Just as with any hospital birth plan, it is unlikely that a family will have access to all their wishes. By exploring the many options provided here, a family, together with their birth team, can identify one or two key needs in the event of an HBC and advocate for those items before consenting to a cesarean. Plan C is not meant to be handed to doctors and nurses. Rather it is kept in a woman's chart as a reminder about the family's surgical birth desires.

Directions for use:

1. Beginning with the "Before the cesarean" section, circle the bulleted option(s) you would like to have during a surgical birth. Feel free to add any additional items.

2. Review the items you have circled and, from those points, identify one or two non-negotiables. Write those in the Summary section.

3. Considering what you have circled and what is in your heart when you think about your ideal birth, list what your key needs and highest intentions are for a surgical birth. For example, your key needs may be that you are able to hold your baby in the OR and your highest inten-

tion might be that your body is treated with respect and at the baby's sex is not announced.

Summary

Non-negotiable options before consenting to a cesarean:

_____

_____

_____

Key needs for a cesarean:

_____

_____

_____

Highest intention for a surgical birth:

_____

_____

_____

Before the cesarean

- I would like a few minutes alone with my partner before consenting to a cesarean / before leaving for the operating room.

- I want to meet and speak with the OB who will be performing my surgery.

- I request both my partner and midwife/doula to provide support in the OR.

- If I do not have an epidural, I would like to walk to the OR.

- I do not want medical residents in the OR during my birth.

- If I require IV antibiotics, I want them to be given post-cord clamping so my baby does not receive the antibiotics.

In the OR—Mother

- I request that all staff in the OR introduce themselves and say hello to my baby.

- I would like a moment of silence in the OR before the surgery begins.

- I understand that trembling is normal and I do not want to be given anti-shaking medications.

- Do not tie my arms down.

- Keep casual conversation outside the OR.

- I want my support person to take photos in the OR.

- I would like a mirror so I can watch the birth of my baby.

- I would like the screen lowered as my baby is being born.

- I want to keep my placenta. If you need to send my placenta to the lab, take a small sample and leave the rest for me. Do not put my placenta in any preservatives.

- I prefer suturing over staples and request a clear bandage like Suture Strip Plus over my entire incision rather than Steri-Strips. I understand that using sutures may shorten my healing time and possibly result in a more cosmetically appealing scar.

In the OR—Baby

- I request immediate skin-to-skin contact.

- Do not bathe, clean, swaddle, or footprint my baby.

- I want to begin breastfeeding in the OR.

- I request delayed cord cutting.

- I want my partner to cut the baby's cord after it is done pulsing.

Reminders for the partner in the OR and after the birth

- Pull down your mask, smile, kiss me, tell me I am strong.

- Only wear a scrubs overcoat, not a shirt, so our baby can be skin-to-skin with you.

- Tell me what is happening during the surgery / remain quiet during the birth unless I ask a question.

- Stay with the baby. Keep your hand on the baby. Talk to the baby. Insist on holding our baby.

- Do not introduce our baby to family or friends. I want that privilege.

- If our baby is in the NICU, do not show me pictures. Do not share pictures with anyone. If our baby is in the NICU, take a lot of pictures and videos.

- Do not text or email photos or post about the birth on social media without checking with me first.

Postpartum support network in the hospital

Call _____ to take care of the children at home.

Call _____ to take care of our pets.

Call _____ to bring what we need from home.

Call _____ to start our meal train at the hospital / when we get home.

Call _____ to clean our home before we are discharged.

Postpartum support network at home

Call _____ to meet us at home when we are discharged.

Call _____ to stay with me during the day.

Call _____ to stay with me during the night.

Call _____ to help with childcare of older siblings.

Call _____ to help with our pets.

Call _____ to pick up groceries and supplies.

Call _____ to help with household chores.

Call _____ to keep me company.

APPENDIX B:
CARING FOR THE HBC MOTHER:
INFORMATION FOR PARTNERS AND SUPPORT PEOPLE

When a planned out-of-hospital becomes a homebirth cesarean, the support of the partner or a trusted other person is essential in helping the mother with physical, emotional, and mental healing.

Physical care

Following a cesarean birth, the mom will need a support person to stay with her throughout the day and night for the first week or two, to help her get up and move around, to assist the baby, and to ensure that the mom has food, water, and comfort items nearby.

In the early days at home, the new mom will remain resting and may only get up to stretch, use the toilet, and shower.

Sleep is important for the mom's physical and mental wellbeing, and it will speed her recovery process. Providing extra pillows, a quiet environment, and encouragement to rest will allow the mom to get the sleep she needs.

The mother will need someone to prepare nutritious, fiber-rich meals and snacks for her, and to have these available to her throughout the day and night.

HBC mothers need plenty of fluids to stay hydrated, to build their milk supply, and to help with healing. The support person should ensure that the mother always has a full water bottle.

Most mothers need help getting out of bed, walking, and stepping into the shower. If there are stairs in the home, she may need to sleep downstairs until she can comfortably climb stairs. If the bed is high off the ground or too low, she may want to sleep in a recliner or on the couch for some time.

Many mothers are frustrated by their lack of mobility in the early days, and will need reminders to prioritize rest and time with the baby, rather than diaper changing, cooking, cleaning, or hosting guests.

Managing pain
After discharge from the hospital, the mom will need help managing her pain medications. When post-surgical moms are exhausted, waking around the clock, and groggy from narcotics, they may find it confusing to keep track of which medications to take, the dosages, and the frequency.

Partners and support people can help by ensuring that they themselves are clear on the pain relief regimen given by the physician prior to hospital discharge, and that they have the doctor's phone number in case of questions.

At home, the partner or support person can remind the mom when to take her medications and write down when she took them. The mother should be encouraged to take her medications before her pain is intolerable. If she waits too long it can be difficult to control her pain, since medications take time to become effective.

The mom will be unable to drive until she is no longer using narcotic pain medication and can easily press the pedals in the car without pain or hesitation. This can be two or more weeks after birth.

Emotional care
For many partners, it can be shocking how exhausted the mother is after an HBC. The cesarean birth itself is a huge drain on a woman's resources, and she is still making the physical transition through pregnancy, birth, and into postpartum recovery that any birthing woman would experience. Along with the exhaustion that the mom feels, she is beginning to process the events of her birth, as well as feeding and building a relationship with her baby. These tasks are incredibly demanding on her body and mind, and she will need ample support as she works her way through the maze of emotions.

After the frequent interruption and lack of privacy in the hospital, many women need the home to be quiet, calm, and private in the early weeks. Even trusted friends and family members may bother her, yet she may be unable to communicate her reluctance to have visitors. Partners can clarify who, if anyone, is welcome to visit and can update others on ways they can still provide support for the new family.

Partners and support people can create a safe opportunity for healing by guarding mom's emotional wellbeing, listening to her when she needs to talk, and acknowledging her complicated emotions. A support person should listen openly, without judgment or the need to falsely reassure. Some women need to process the birth by recounting details, impressions, and feelings many, many times.

It can be hard for partners to truly listen when they have their own mourning about the birth, or when the mother has negative feelings about the role the partner played in the birth. In these cases, the mother and partner can identify a supportive listener who is willing to sit with the mother and hear her story. It can also be helpful for the partner to seek the support of a friend, relative, or mental health professional who can empathetically listen to the partner's own story and emotions.

The partner may also need a break from being at home with the mother and will appreciate a chance to meet a friend for coffee, or talk on the phone while the mom is resting. When partners are well cared for by others, they can provide the loving support that mothers need.

HBC women often feel like they failed at giving birth, and they may need frequent reassurance and encouragement from those around them that they did a great job in birthing and caring for the baby and that they are strong mothers.

Supporting mom's mental health

Women who experience an HBC may be at a higher risk of suffering from postpartum mood and anxiety disorders, including depression and anxiety. Post-traumatic stress disorder (PTSD) can also be common after a traumatic birth.

The partner or main support person has the unique perspective of witnessing a mother's mental wellbeing across the days, weeks, and months following birth, and he or she can offer valuable insight to the mom's healthcare providers. In many cases, the mother herself has no reference point for knowing if what she is feeling is normal, and she may not be aware that she needs further assessment. The partner/support person should attend postpartum appointments with the mother to help the birth team understand how the mother is coping emotionally.

Partners and trusted support people must watch the mom for signs of postpartum mood and anxiety disorders. They can often spot signs that the mom is struggling even before she herself realizes she is suffering. They can ask the birth team what the signs and symptoms are for postpartum mood and anxiety disorders and request referrals for local mental health professionals and national mental health support.

The partner or support person must be unafraid to ask the mom if she is concerned about her mental health. If the mom expresses worry or if the partner feels concerned about her mental health, the partner/support person should encourage the mom to get screened for mood and anxiety disorders by her midwife, physician, or a mental health professional.

If the mom seems to be considering endangering herself or the baby, seek professional help immediately. Contact the local emergency room; the mom's hospital physician, midwife, or mental health professional; or the 24 hour National Suicide Prevention Lifeline 1-800-273-8255.

Help around the home
After a surgical birth, the mother will not be able to cook, clean, or do other household chores for at least the first few weeks. New parents are almost always surprised by the amount of time it takes just to care for the baby, and cleaning and laundry seem like insurmountable tasks at first. Because the mom is recovering from major abdominal surgery, her fatigue will be compounded by physical, mental, and emotion strains.

Even a few weeks after the birth, HBC mothers continue to be exhausted and sore, and they are just beginning to resume some of their normal home activities. When the partner returns to work, the mother will still need help with cooking, cleaning, and caring for the baby and older children. Her stamina will still be low, and she will need to nap daily to be able to continue healing.

When the mother is unable to help with the household work, it can be exhausting for the partner to be responsible for taking care of her, the baby, the household, and other children at home. Consider enlisting the support of trusted family, friends, and neighbors who can relieve some of the burden, and allow the partner more time to be with the mother and rest. Helpers should be reminded ahead of time that the mother will be tired and may not want to socialize, and that she might not feel comfortable with others holding the baby just yet.

It can be helpful to consider hiring a postpartum doula to help out at home and assist with caring for the baby. Local midwifery schools and doula training programs can give referrals for low-cost or free postpartum doulas.

APPENDIX C:

RESOURCES FOR HBC MOTHERS AND FAMILIES

HBC support

Online and in-person healing retreats for mothers who experienced a homebirth cesarean.

www.CourtneyJarecki.com

In 2011 Courtney Jarecki created a closed Facebook support group for HBC mothers and birth professionals. Search "Homebirth Cesarean" on Facebook and request permission to join if you are an HBC mother or a birth professional.

The Homebirth Cesarean website offers HBC birth stories, photo galleries, and resources.

www.HomeBirthCesarean.com

Homebirth Cesarean: Stories and Support for Families and Healthcare Providers
Written by: Courtney Key Jarecki with Laurie Perron Mednick, CPM.
A comprehensive resource for families and birth professionals as they navigate pregnancy, homebirth cesarean, and the postpartum.

Healing from a Homebirth Cesarean: A companion workbook for mothers who planned an out-of-hospital birth that ended in the operating room
Written by: Courtney Key Jarecki
A powerful and innovative approach, to align the cognitive, physical, emotional, and relational areas of life affected by a homebirth cesarean.

General Cesarean Support

International Cesarean Awareness Network (ICAN) works to improve maternal-child health by preventing unnecessary cesareans through education, providing support for cesarean recovery, and promoting vaginal birth after cesarean (VBAC).
www.ican-online.org

Birth Trauma Support

Birthing from Within offers private birth story-listening sessions to help heal from difficult births.
www.birthingfromwithin.com

> *When Survivors Give Birth: Understanding and Healing the Effects of*
> *Early Sexual Abuse on Childbearing Women*
> Written by: Penny Simkin and Phyllis Klaus

> *Waking the Tiger: Healing Trauma*
> Written by: Peter A. Levine with Ann Frederick

> *Traumatic Birth*
> Written by: Cheryl Tatano Beck, Jeanne Watson Driscoll, and Sue Watson

Perinatal Mood and Anxiety Disorder Support for Mothers

National Alliance on Mental Health provides state-by-state hotlines for women.
www.nami.org

Postpartum Progress provides community and information for women.
www.postpartumprogress.com

Postpartum Support International increases awareness among public and professional communities about the emotional changes that women experience during pregnancy and postpartum.
www.postpartum.net

Postpartum Stress Center provides support, counseling, and education to women and their families who experience difficulties related to pregnancy, pregnancy loss, and the postpartum period.
www.postpartumstress.com

National Suicide Prevention Lifeline helps individuals in suicidal crisis within the United States. A trained counselor will answer the phone 24/7.
1-800-273-8255
www.suicidepreventionlifeline.org

> *This Isn't What I Expected: Overcoming Postpartum Depression*
> Written by: Karen Kleiman

> *What Am I Thinking? Having a Baby after Postpartum Depression*
> Written by: Karen Kleiman

Postpartum Mood and Anxiety Disorder Support for Partners
Postpartum Dads help families overcome postpartum depression.
www.postpartumdads.org

> *The Postpartum Husband: Practical Solutions for Living with Postpartum Depression*
> Written by: Karen Kleiman

Uterus, Scar, and Body Healing: Information and Practitioner Location
International Pelvic Pain Society
www.pelvicpain.org

The Pacific Center for Pelvic Pain and Dysfunction
www.jmweissmd.com

The Upledger Institute for CranioSacral Therapy
www.upledger.com

Arvigo Therapy for Maya Abdominal Therapy and Spiritual Healing
www.arvigotherapy.com

National Certification Commission for Acupuncture and Oriental Medicine
www.nccaom.org

Myofascial Release
www.myofascialrelease.com

>*Wild Feminine: Finding Power, Spirit & Joy in the Female Body*
>Written by: Tami Lynn Kent
>Holistic approach to regaining power, joy, and love for your body by restoring balance in the pelvic bowl.

Probiotics & Gut Health

Blood-type formulated probiotics
www.dadamo.com/article_bloodtype_probiotic.htm

Vaginal ecology probiotics
www.vitanica.com
www.integrativepro.com

Breastfeeding

La Leche League International is an international organization with local links for mother-to-mother breastfeeding support, encouragement, information, and education.
www.llli.org

Information, support, and online forum for mothers experiencing low milk production, and online resource for healthcare providers who help mothers breastfeed.
www.lowmilksupply.org

>*The Breastfeeding Mother's Guide to Making More Milk*
>Written by: Diana West, BA, IBCLC, and Lisa Marasco, MA, IBCLC

Milk Sharing

Human Milk Banking Association of North America provides links to milk banks throughout the United States and Canada, information about how to donate or obtain milk, guidelines for safe milk banking, and additional resources.
www.hmbana.org

Resource for the safety, mechanisms, and informed choice process of community-based milk sharing.
www.eatsonfeets.org
www.hm4hb.net

Parenting Resources

Hand in Hand Parenting provides parents with the insights and skills they need to listen to and connect with their children in a way that allows each child to thrive.
www.handinhandparenting.org

Kelly Mom provides evidence-based information and community connections around parenting, child development, and breastfeeding.
www.kellymom.com

Re-Evaluation Counseling to exchange effective help with each other in order to free themselves from the effects of past distress experiences.
www.rc.org

APPENDIX D:

SCHEDULE OF MENTAL HEALTH, TRANSPORT, AND CESAREAN TOPICS

These topics are to be integrated with other standard prenatal conversations.

First Trimester

- Begin the discussion of hospital transport and interventions in the hospital, including cesarean.

- Ensure that both the mother and her partner understand the payment plan in the event of a transport and a cesarean.

- Provide local and national mental health resources and ask mental health screening questions.

Second Trimester

- Ask the mother to research which hospital is her best choice (location, insurance, established relationships with providers, services, etc.) and report back at the next appointment.

- Discuss childbirth class options that include transport and cesarean education.

- At the 16- or 20-week solo visit, review the confidentiality worksheet with the mother, giving her the opportunity to discuss sensitive information about past or current abuse (physical, emotional, or sexual), past trauma, and past and current mental health. Make referrals as needed.

- Provide the Plan C worksheet and ask the family to complete it and bring it to their 28- or 32- week appointment. Ask that the partner and all support people attending the birth to be at this appointment to review Plan C.

- Ask mental health screening questions and discuss the spectrum of PMADs, postpartum PTSD, and their symptoms. Ensure that the partner/support person is at this appointment.

- Recommend taking a hospital tour and report back at the next visit.

Third Trimester

- Refer to Plan C at the 36-week visit, discuss a clear strategy for deciding which members of the birth team should plan to accompany the mom to the hospital, and how/by whom postpartum care will be conducted in the event of a cesarean.

- Advise the mother to pack a bag for the hospital, including items for herself, her partner, and the baby.

- Review postpartum support and care for both vaginal and cesarean birth. Refer to Plan C. Provide handouts of local and national cesarean resources.

- Request that the partner print a map and directions from home/birth center to the hospital, advise the partner to practice the drive from home/birth center to hospital, install the infant car seat and have it inspected.

- Screen with mental health questions and mention the standard screening worksheet she will receive postpartum regardless of her birth outcome.

APPENDIX E:

SCREENING TOOLS

The Postpartum Stress Center provides support, counseling, and education to women and their families. On their website are several assessment tools that all birth professionals can use in their practice with pregnant and postpartum women.[25] Below is a summary of some of these tools, that mothers can use for themselves and birth professionals can provide to clients.

Screening with questions

The Postpartum Stress Center provides a list of assessment questions that should be asked of every woman, regardless of her clinical presentation. Some simple yet powerful questions include:

- Do you have a history of depression?

- Is there anything you are afraid to tell me but think I should know?

- Are you worried about the way you feel right now?

- If you are physically or emotionally struggling with breastfeeding, how important is continuing to you?

---

25 www.postpartumstress.com/professional-development/assessments/

The Edinburgh Postnatal Depression Scale (EPDS)

The EPDS is a clinically validated screening tool for birth professionals. The Postpartum Stress Center recommends that healthcare professionals working with the perinatal population use the EPDS as an integral part of their assessment for depression. This is a 10-item assessment tool that is valid and reliable for detecting postpartum depression. It is user-friendly, easy to administer, and easy to score. A score of 10-12 is considered the cut off for PPD and women with that score or higher should be referred for further evaluation or treatment.

Assessment questions include:

I have felt scared or panicky for no good reason.

3   Yes, often
2   Yes, sometimes
1   No, not much
0   No, not at all

Things have been too much for me.

3   Yes, most of the time I haven't been able to cope at all.
2   Yes, sometimes I haven't been coping as well as usual.
1   No, most of the time I have coped well.
0   No, I have been coping as well as ever.

The Postpartum Distress Measure (PDM)

The PDM can be used as a conversation starter for women to begin pulling apart the many layers of emotions that come with pregnancy, birth, and becoming a mother. The 10 questions reference the past week, including the day the woman is filling out the assessment. The PDM has yet to be validated in clinical trials.

Questions include:

I am crying more than usual.

0   This is true most of the time.
1   This is true some of the time.
2   This is true only occasionally.
3   No, this is not true.

I'm afraid I will never feel better.

0   This is true most of the time.
1   This is true some of the time.
2   This is true only occasionally.
3   No, this is not true.

Develop your own screening tool

Screening assessments only work if they are used. If birth professionals are more comfortable creating their own set of questions, they can look further into the assessments provided here and customize them to fit their individual practices.

Birth professionals must be asking their screening questions with every woman regardless of her history, current emotional state, and birth outcome. If a woman appears to be suffering from a PMAD or PTSD, a birth professional's job is to validate, reassure, and provide her with professional mental health resources.

APPENDIX F:

INCISION CARE AND HEALING AFTER AN HBC

Your midwife or the surgeon who attended your cesarean birth, may have specific care guidelines based upon your individual health and healing. While you may seek care from your midwife for general postpartum issues, it is important to also contact your surgeon if you are having complications with your incision.

Incision care: Closures and dressings
After you give birth, your skin incision will be stapled, glued, or stitched with dissolving sutures. Be sure to clarify which type of closure you have prior to discharge.

If your incision is sutured, you will probably have a wide dressing placed over the entire wound. While the dressing is on, you will need to keep the area clean and dry.

If your doctor used staples on your incision, they will usually be removed prior to discharge from the hospital, and vertical bandages may be placed on the incision afterward. Keeping these vertical bandages on as long as possible can reduce scarring and help maintain tissue integrity. If you want to remove the bandages before they naturally fall off, doing that in the shower, while warm water runs over them, will be the most comfortable.

An incision that was glued can be gently washed with warm water and patted dry.

Incision warning signs
You may notice slight drainage of fluid from the incision site for the first few days. If this drainage increases or becomes pussy or bloody, contact your physician.

Stitches and staples can cause irritation, bruising, redness, swelling, itching, or numbness. This is normal, and should begin to decrease as stitches dissolve or soon after staples are removed.

Infection
Tips for reducing the risk of infection:

- If you have a dressing over the incision, change it if it gets wet or soiled.

- Wait to shower until at least three days after birth, and wait seven days to take a bath.

- Do not scrub or rub the incision.

- Do not use lotion or powder on the incision until after it is fully closed.

Signs of infection
Call your doctor if you notice any of the following:

- A yellow or green discharge.

- A change in the odor of the discharge.

- The incision appears larger or puffier than before.

- Redness or hardening of the surrounding area.

- The incision is hot to the touch.

- Fever over 100.4 degrees Fahrenheit. Be aware that Tylenol is a fever reducer and it can be harder to detect a fever if it is used.

- Increasing or unusual pain.

- Excessive bleeding that has soaked through the dressing.

Pain medications

The healing process from an HBC varies greatly from woman to woman. While some women rely on pain medications for only the first week, others need pain relievers for two weeks or more. If you have concerns about your pain levels or your need for medication, contact your physician or midwife.

Narcotic pain relievers may cause you to feel groggy or disoriented, and you may have a harder time rousing from sleep. Ensure that a support person is nearby at all times in the first week after returning home from the hospital so that he or she can attend to the needs of the baby while you rest. You will not be able to drive a car until you are no longer using narcotic pain medications and your are pain free enough to firmly press the brake pedal without hesitation.

Some women find that in addition to the pain medication prescribed by their doctor, taking the homeopathic *Bellis perennis* can help with the soreness, bruising, and swelling from the surgery. You can find this in small pellet form at natural food stores, and it is safe to take while using other medications and breastfeeding. The recommended dose is 200C, taken one to three times daily, and away from food or drink other than water. You can ask about other natural pain relief from naturopathic doctors or at your local natural food store.

Bowel health and nutrition

Many women suffer from painful gas, bloating, and constipation following a cesarean. The digestive system slows during labor and birth, plus narcotics and anesthesia can make digestive problems worse. If your midwife or doctor prescribed an iron supplement, consider waiting until your digestion returns to normal before taking iron, which can cause constipation.

Your care provider may recommend a stool softener to begin taking soon after birth. Vitamin C acts as a mild laxative and can be taken in tablet or powdered form up to 3000mg daily. You can begin taking 1000mg daily, and increase the amount by 500mg until it produces comfortable bowel movements but not enough to cause diarrhea. Vitamin C is safe to take with breastfeeding and can be continued until bowels regain their normal motility, sometimes as long as six weeks after a cesarean birth.

As soon as you are able, begin getting out of bed and gently moving and walking every few hours throughout the day to help bowel function. A warm heating pad or hot water bottle on the abdomen can also relieve painful gas.

Eating small, easily digested, high-fiber meals with plenty of water can help. Avoid starchy, white foods, which are often nutrient poor and can add to constipation. You will need plenty of high-fiber, iron-rich foods to help your bowel motility and rebuild your hemoglobin levels. The increased blood loss from surgery means that iron stores are low, making anemia very common. Ask your helpers to prepare salads with dark, leafy greens such as arugula, kale, or spinach, which can be combined with apples or dried cranberries and sunflower or pumpkin seeds for a healthy meal. Instead of carbonated and cold drinks, choose warm drinks such as peppermint or fennel tea, water, or other clear fluids.

Basic movement

Moving around and caring for yourself and your baby will be challenging in the first weeks following a cesarean birth. When getting out of bed, rising from a chair, or using stairs, you may feel stretching or tugging at the incision site. This is normal. You will not harm the incision site with slow, gentle movements. You can hold a pillow or rolled towel against the incision when rolling over, sitting up, or even walking. This stabilization tool, braced against the incision site, can also be used when coughing, sneezing, laughing, or crying. Abdominal splinting is another option to help brace the incision site.

Walking and moving around your home, while uncomfortable, can be beneficial for your healing and circulation, reduce the risk of clotting in your legs, and helps help your organs shift back into place. After a few weeks, as your stamina returns, you can start walking around your neighborhood to help with both your physical and mental wellbeing. Remember to listen to your body's signals, including fatigue and discomfort, to guide the amount of activity you do in the first months after birth. Refrain from abdominal restoration exercises until your incision is fully healed.

Do not lift anything heavier than your baby for the first few weeks. You will not be able to do household chores such as laundry, cooking, and cleaning, so you will need a helper to do these tasks until you are healed and comfortable when moving around. Activities such as vacuuming and hanging laundry will pull on your incision and you must refrain from these movements in the first few weeks.

Gently begin touching your incision site when you feel emotionally and physically ready and it is no longer painful. Touching your incision can alert you to complications such as a hematoma, which is a hard clot of blood in the tissue beneath the incision. Touching your incision can be emotionally charged for many women; however, this gentle attention may help you begin to process your birth experience.

APPENDIX G:

BREASTFEEDING AFTER A HOMEBIRTH CESAREAN

Breastfeeding your baby after a homebirth cesarean can be a rewarding and possibly overwhelming undertaking. In addition to exhaustion, physical healing, and the emotional turbulence from the birth, you will need to balance the differing opinions and advice from nurses, your birth team, lactation consultants, and physicians. It can be helpful to identify one of those people you trust the most, and ask her to help. Most importantly, trust your intuition to guide your decision-making as you begin to nourish your baby.

Any amount of breastmilk your baby receives is valuable for her health, but the choice to continue to breastfeed is ultimately yours. In deciding to continue to breastfeed, you must take into account your own mental, emotional, and physical health. If the thought of breastfeeding after your HBC feels staggering, that's okay. You have to do what is best for you.

Many women feel guilty if they are unable to breastfeed. Seek positive encouragement for the hard work you did to birth your baby and feed her, regardless of the route!

Getting started in the operating room

- Once your baby is born, if you are both stable in the operating room, your partner or nurse may lay him across your chest to allow him to latch. Your nurse or partner will remain close by to keep the baby safe on your chest, since you will be groggy and your arms may be restrained. Even if your baby just nuzzles and licks at the breast, he will benefit from being held close to you, which will regulate his body temperature and breathing. It can be helpful to discuss this with your doctor and nurses prior to the birth, and clarify your hopes and needs for breastfeeding as soon as possible.

- Even if you do not feel ready to breastfeed, you can ask the nurse to place your baby skin-to-skin on you, and cover both of you with a warm blanket to help your baby maintain her body temperature.

- You can request that the nurses refrain from washing or vigorously drying off your baby. The smell of amniotic fluid on her skin mimics the smell of colostrum, and helps her initiate nursing when she can smell the fluid on her own hands. Also, many HBC mothers feel that when their babies were washed immediately after birth, they lost an important scent connection.

- If your baby cannot remain with you after the birth, your partner can act as your advocate and let the hospital staff know that being reunited with your baby is your priority, that you plan to breastfeed as soon as possible, and that you do not wish the baby to be given supplemental formula or a pacifier.

In the recovery room

- If you were not able to begin nursing in the operating room, you can begin as soon as you and the baby are stable. In some cases, the hospital staff might need reminders that you must hold your baby, and that routine interventions and procedures can be done with the baby at your breast.

- Skin-to-skin contact will help keep your baby calm, boost your milk production, and will help him begin nursing. Ask the nurses for assistance getting into a comfortable position, and use plenty of pillows to keep your baby in a good position.

- During the initial feeding, don't be overly concerned about getting a perfect latch or position. If you can find a position where you are at ease and your baby can freely access your breasts, you can both enjoy these moments. In fact, many HBC moms find that they are the most comfortable when nursing immediately after the birth, since the anesthesia still provides good pain relief. Enjoy these moments with your baby.

- It can be helpful to remind nurses that you are letting your baby guide her first feeding, and you will ask for help if you need it. Sometimes nurses are overly eager to assist in positioning the baby at the breast, and this can feel degrading or disempowering for some women.

- During this time partners often begin taking photos, calling family members, and posting social media updates about the birth. Let your partner know if you prefer to spend this time privately as a family, or if photos and phone calls are okay.

- Remind others that this first feeding is a sacred moment for you, and ask your partner to help keep the room quiet, dimly lit, and warm.

- Visitors should be delayed until after you have nursed your baby and rested.

When mom and baby are separated

- Ask the nurse for an immediate consultation with a lactation consultant to help you formulate a breastfeeding plan.

- Request that a breast pump be brought into your room so that you can begin pumping as soon as possible. This will help your milk come in sooner.

- It can often be difficult to pump colostrum. Hand expressing this milk is a useful skill that your lactation consultant can teach you. This can be used in combination with mechanical pumping.

- Make sure that your baby has an item of clothing that you have worn, and that you have a blanket or hat from your baby. Breastfeeding is an intensely scent-oriented process, and this can help both of you feel more connected and increase your oxytocin levels.

- Remind your partner how/if you want to receive updates from the NICU. Some mothers cannot bear to hear that others are taking care of and holding the baby, while others want all information shared with them. You can also ask your partner to refrain from posting baby announcements, photos, and updates until you have had the chance to meet and be reunited with your baby.

While in the hospital

- Request that a lactation consultant visit you as soon as possible after your surgical birth to help establish a solid breastfeeding relationship and answer your questions.

- After all surgical births, regardless of the status of the nursing relationship, ask the lactation consultant to bring a breast pump to your room and have her demonstrate how to use it properly. She can give you advice on how often to pump, how long to pump, and how to coordinate the pumping with nursing your baby.

- Performing breast massage and hand expression frequently the first few days between pumpings will help bring your milk in.

- Because of the medications given throughout a cesarean birth, increased blood loss, longer separation times from your baby, and a sleepier baby, it is common for your milk to be delayed coming in by an additional day or two. Many lactation consultants recommend that cesarean mothers begin pumping within eight hours of birth to help bring their milk in as soon as possible. You can continue pumping every few hours, along with nursing at the breast, until you feel confident in your milk supply.

- Droplets of colostrum collected during pumping or hand expressing can be fed to your baby with a feeding syringe, spoon, or supplemental nurser (a small flexible tube taped to the breast while nursing).

- Your baby will be weighed daily while you are in the hospital. Due to the amount of IV fluids you received during birth, she may be born with extra fluid, which causes her weight to be higher than it would otherwise. This extra water is excreted in the first few days, leading to additional weight loss. Keep this in mind if hospital staff are mentioning too much weight loss.

- As anesthesia begins to wear off, many mothers will become more uncomfortable. Experiment with different nursing positions until you find what works for you and your baby. The football hold and side-lying nursing (with the head of the bed elevated) can help reduce the pressure over your incision. Your nurse, midwife, or doula can help you learn these breastfeeding positions. Do not feel obligated to use specific nursing positions if they don't work for you and your baby.

- Placing a pillow against your incision when nursing protects your incision if your baby kicks. Nursing pillows usually don't work well after a cesarean birth since they put too much pressure on the incision.

- Ask your nurse to clarify your instructions and timing for pain medication, and ask her to remind you when it is time to take more. She can write down what you are taking and reassure you that it is safe and compatible with breastfeeding.

- While your baby is receiving small droplets of colostrum in the first few days, the amount of pain medication he receives is minimal, but it may still make him a bit groggy. You might need to rouse your baby by unwrapping him, changing his diaper, or rubbing his feet to keep him actively sucking at your breast.

- Friends and family members must be reminded that your sole focus is on recovering from surgical birth and feeding your baby, not entertaining guests or handing the baby to others to hold.

- Enlist your partner's help in tracking your nursing frequency and the baby's urination and bowel movements. This can be a great way for partners to engage with the baby and support the breastfeeding relationship.

At home with the baby

- Ensure that your partner has lined up adequate support for you and your household in the early weeks postpartum. You will be unable to do housework, cooking, and childcare for older children for at least the first few weeks while your incision heals and your strength returns.

You and your partner will be exhausted from the sleepless nights, and housekeeping and preparing meals will be daunting. You need extra help.

- When arriving home, it can be helpful for you to recreate the babymoon you lost while in the hospital. You and your baby can get into bed and remain skin-to-skin for the first several days at home. This babymoon is helpful for bonding, building a strong milk supply, and allowing rest for both of you. You will need your partner or other helpful family member or friend to check in often, bring food and water, and assist with changing the baby's diaper.

- If your milk seems delayed coming in, consult with your midwife or lactation consultant. She may advise you to nurse more frequently, continue pumping between feedings, or take milk-producing herbs and supplements.

- If your baby's weight loss is a concern, you can request to borrow a baby scale from your midwife or lactation consultant to weigh your baby between appointments. This can prevent you and your baby from needing to be driven to an appointment just for a weight check.

- If your baby needs more milk than you are producing, your midwife or lactation consultant can recommend other milk supplements, including donor breast milk available through a milk bank, hospital, or a casual milk-sharing community. Homemade or commercial formula are also options.

APPENDIX H:

PHYSICAL HEALING MODALITIES AFTER AN HBC

Here we offer an overview of four alternative healing modalities that HBC mothers and birth professionals have recommended for optimal physical healing. There are more pathways to healing than we can mention here, but if a modality resonates with you, see the resource list in Appendix C for a reference on how to locate providers in your area.

Splinting or binding

Women often store their emotional pain between the rib cage and pelvis, says Kelly Dean, a physical therapist specializing in abdominal rehabilitation. "If there was miscarriage, infertility, birth trauma, or anything related to femininity and sexuality, it's stored in that area. After birth, women tend to bury their painful emotions in their pelvis as a survival technique because they need to focus on their baby." Dean says that if a mother emotionally disconnects from her body and does not address her mental well-being, a whole chain of physical events can happen that can lead to muscle compensation, pain, and pelvic floor problems.

Splinting, also known as binding, is a technique that can be used as early as 24-hours after surgery, or even years later, to knit the abdominal muscle fibers back together, and help with emotional healing. Splinting the core pulls the entire body together, restores balance, and is the first step to physical healing after a surgical birth.

> I never would have known to even ask for a splint if my midwives didn't bring it to me. Without it, I felt like my insides were pouring out and like the lines between my body and the rest of the world were blurred. Wearing it, I felt contained and stronger, with better energetic boundaries.
> —RACHEL (2009/HBC, WESTERN U.S.)

There are several binding options to choose from to accommodate body shapes, as well as comfort and flexibility. Soft splints are great for women soon after birth and tend to be the most comfortable. Firmer splints are rigid and fit more snugly, providing more core stability. If purchasing an abdominal splint, women should choose a splint they can wear during waking hours and ideally overnight as well. Splints should be worn over an undershirt to limit skin irritation. Women can also use a Moby wrap or a long scarf to bind their bellies.

Splinting is a temporary healing modality, one that shouldn't be used for longer than six weeks, depending on the severity of abdominal separation. When a woman finds she no longer wants to wear the splint or feels like it isn't helping anymore, it should be discontinued.

Core and scar care
Bryan Baisinger, DC treats women for complications after cesarean such as numbness or discomfort around the incision, painful sex, incontinence, low back pain, pelvis issues, and gait anomalies. "Usually cesarean mothers have a partially deactivated lower core that is unable to fully engage," says Baisinger. "This is due to pregnancy stretching the muscles of the abdomen and surgery separating those already compromised muscles. These women are performing abdomen exercises and other physical activities but they aren't seeing results."

In addition to abdominal muscles that can't fully engage, adhesions, also known as internal scar tissue, form masses between organs, muscles, and fascia. Adhesions can be found between the uterus and bladder, an ovary and adjacent muscle, and anywhere around the incision sites. Adhesions may be painful or may go unnoticed and usually lead to altered strength and motion patterns of the body possibly resulting in low back, hip, and/or pelvic pain.

Regardless of the internal situation, many women seek treatment to help the external scar become less noticeable. A red scar indicates that circulation is present, while a white scar means circulation has shut down. When a scar is elevated and feels like a bobby pin or has keloid formation, treatment once the incision is fully closed, usually after six weeks, can help minimize its appearance.

For women who want to improve the integrity of their scar while also soft-ening adhesions, Baisinger recommends myofascial release, a protocol of gentle stretching around the scar tissue, in combination with therapeutic ultrasound, and very light *guasha*, which is light rubbing with a blunt handheld tool in the area of the scar. This brings blood to the area for additional healing and possible nerve regeneration. Therapeutic ultrasound can be helpful in breaking up excess material that has built up around the scar. This allows for freer movement and circulation, and it reduces adhesions.

> *My scar and the skin around it felt tight, like a sunburn. Plus, I was numb from halfway down my vulva to almost my bellybutton. There was no feeling at all—I could have cut myself and not known. I started rolling the scar between my fingers, pressing and kneading until it was bordering between uncomfortable and painful. As I worked on it, the length of my scar increased and my "c-shelf" became more of a gradual slope than an abrupt shelf. Where my scar had started out very tight and bound up in the layers beneath, it became longer, looser, and free from some of the adhesions.*
> —Leah (2012/HBC, Western U.S.)

Pelvic floor work

Specially trained care providers can offer women a healing modality called pelvic floor work to help restore alignment of the pelvic muscles and or-gans affected by pregnancy and birth. Pelvic floor work utilizes intervaginal trigger point work to help women regain their pelvic bowl integrity.

Women's health physical therapist Tami Lynn Kent adds in fascial and energy work to her pelvic floor practice, thus offering a unique healing experience for women called Holistic Pelvic Care™. She describes this work as encompassing "the fascia and muscles of the pelvic floor and also the ovaries and the womb—the whole creative center of a woman." Kent works on realigning the pelvis physically and energetically to enhance the flow of pelvic energy and restore the pelvic bowl.

> *During my pelvic floor work sessions, grief and failure were released from my muscle memory without re-traumatizing me. I connected my energetic womb love to my daughter.*
> —Sue (2010/HBC, Western U.S.)

Maya Abdominal Therapy

Maya abdominal therapy is an external, non-invasive massage-like technique that guides abdominal organs to their proper position. In pregnancy, organs naturally shift to accommodate the growing baby. During a cesarean, the uterus may be removed from the body cavity and re-inserted after the baby is born. Maya abdominal therapy helps realign the internal map of the body. Some Maya abdominal therapists combine spiritual and energetic work along with traditional physical manipulations to help the body heal from trauma.

Corrine Porterfield, a Maya abdominal practitioner, says, "The somatic work, the act of moving trauma out of the body, helps give people a lifeline and pull them out of their trauma story. A lot of HBC moms experience a disconnection from the pelvis. Energetically, their pelvis or their cesarean scar may feel like an empty space, similar to a vacant closet."

> Two years after my HBC I saw a Maya abdominal practitioner who also used energetic work. I felt like I dropped an emotional 10-pound weight from my pelvis. All the disappointment and failure I was carrying around was suddenly gone.
> —ANN (2011/HBC, MIDWESTERN U.S.)

GLOSSARY

Adhesions: Abnormal connection of tissue, fascia, and organs after surgery. Internal scar tissue.

Back labor: Acute low back pain during contractions, usually due to mal-position of the baby.

Bloody show: Blood-tinged mucus that usually presents in early labor.

Breast crawl: The instinctual ability of newborns to crawl to the mother's breast.

Breech: The position of the baby in which the bottom or feet present first.

Cardinal movements: The typical sequence of fetal positions as the baby descends through the pelvis and vagina.

Constriction ring: A tight band of tissue in the cervix.

C-shelf: Skin that overhangs the cesarean incision due to adhesions, body type, or surgical factors.

Dilation: The opening of the cervix during labor.

Decelerations (decels): A decrease in the fetal heart rate below the baby's baseline.

Epidural: An injection of anesthetic into the space outside the spinal cord.

Fundal height: The measure of the size of the uterus during pregnancy and in the weeks following birth.

Gestational sac: Surrounds the embryo and can be seen via ultrasound in early pregnancy.

Guasha: Traditional Chinese healing practice where the skin is lightly scraped with a blunt object to promote blood flow.

Induction: Any procedure at home or in the hospital used to induce contractions before labor begins on its own.

Keloid: Excessive skin growth within scar tissue that may be painless or extremely painful.

Maya abdominal therapy: Non-invasive technique used to bring the body back into balance by gently repositioning organs that have shifted.

Meconium: Poop formed in-utero that can be passed while baby is still inside the womb or in the first days after birth. Meconium can be concerning if passed in-utero and may be a sign of fetal distress.

Myofascia: The dense, flexible tissue surrounding and covering all muscles and bones.

Placenta previa: Condition where the placenta covers all or part of the cervix.

Postpartum year: The first twelve months after birth.

Pelvic bowl: All the muscles, fascia, and organs contained within the pelvis.

Pelvic floor: The base of the abdomen that is attached to the pelvis.

Special scar: A cesarean scar other than the common low transverse incision.

Splinting: Binding the abdominal muscles to aid in healing abdominal separation.

Steri-Strips: Thin adhesive bandages that pull the skin of an incision together.

Supplemental nurser: A feeding tube device designed to feed a baby at the breast with breast milk or formula.

Therapeutic ultrasound: The use of ultrasound for healing rather than imaging purposes.

Transfer: Pre-labor admittance to the hospital from home.

Transition: The last phase of active labor before pushing.

Transport: Admittance to the hospital during labor.

AUTHOR BIOGRAPHIES

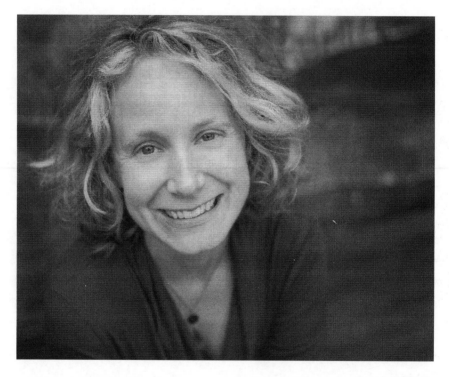

Campbell Salgado

Courtney Key Jarecki has worked as a doula, childbirth educator, and a homebirth midwifery apprentice, but her path forever shifted after the birth of her daughter. In recovering from her 54-hour home labor, hospital transport, and cesarean, Courtney soon began creating a new model of understanding for these types of births, now known as *homebirth cesareans (HBC),* a term she coined. Left without stories that reflected her own journey, she was driven to provide others with resources and support she could not find for herself.

Courtney envisions a future where women of her daughter's generation will birth with knowledge and dignity regardless of location, and in the company of care providers who respect and understand their wishes. She is the founder of the Homebirth Cesarean movement and is actively working to broaden the conversation and education around homebirth cesareans through the support of mothers, families, and birth professionals.

She is also the author of *Healing from a Homebirth Cesarean,* a companion workbook for any mother whose planned out-of-hospital birth ended in the operating room (Incisio Press, 2015).

To attend an in-person or online workshop for birth professionals or a healing retreat for mothers who experienced an HBC, visit www.CourtneyJarecki.com

In balancing her writing, teaching, and leadership activities, she is the mama to Lazadae, wife to Dave, and alpha-female pack leader to hounds Satchel and Maji. She lives in Oregon.

Laurie Perron Mednick has been attending births since 1996, first as a doula and then as a certified professional midwife. Seeking to revise the outdated scripts of birth within midwifery care, Laurie hopes her contribution to this book will challenge other childbirth professionals to broaden their definition of a triumphant birth experience. Laurie adores woodworking and hiking with her husband and three young boys in Washington.

Claudia Baskind's HBC healing journey led her to contribute to this book, to foster greater support for new families and empowered reconsideration for children's experiences. Claudia has facilitated birth healing groups and served as a breastfeeding peer educator. She earned her MFA from the Iowa Writers Workshop and lives in Oregon, where she teaches Connected Parenting classes and enjoys roughhousing with her family.

ACKNOWLEDGEMENTS

There are so many women and men who helped breathe life into *Home-birth Cesarean*. My appreciation for each of you is vast and overflowing.

Thank you, Dave, for creating a situation that allowed me to complete this work while raising our daughter. Satchel, your love, dignified heart, and business savvy kept me warm during so many days of writing on your blue couch. I have deep appreciation and gratitude to the community of donors who rallied around the book concept and supported this endeavor. Thank you, Ann, for your role as the HBC book doula. To the beta readers who took time to provide insight, my deepest gratitude. A huge loving hug to all the mothers, partners, midwives, doulas, and other professionals who believed in my work. And Lazadae, thank you for the gift of your birth. Without you, this wouldn't be.

With much love,

Courtney Key Jarecki

HOMEBIRTH CESAREAN WORKSHOP
AND RETREAT INFORMATION

Workshops for birth professionals

When a woman plans an out-of-hospital birth, or a natural birth in the hospital, she may experience deep grief, trauma, and life-altering mental and emotional outcomes if she ends up in the operating room. The support she receives from her birth team, beginning with her prenatal care and ending with her last postpartum appointment, can influence the next years of her life as a birther, mother, and woman.

These hands-on and interactive workshops are safe havens for birth professionals to learn practical tools and strategies to care for women, families, and themselves during difficult or traumatic births. If you are a seasoned professional, student, or aspiring birth worker, the Homebirth Cesarean workshops will provide you with resources you will call upon many times throughout your career and even in your personal life.

Healing Retreats for HBC mothers

The online, day, and weekend retreat healing circles offer HBC mothers a sacred space, away from the cares of day-to-day life, to pursue a deep healing months or years after a difficult birth. HBC mothers gather with the intention to support each other on a shared quest for knowledge, wisdom, and the reclamation of self.

To learn more about these in-person and online workshops and healing events, please visit: www.CourtneyJarecki.com

Index

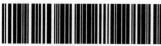

Made in the USA
Lexington, KY
08 February 2017